THERAPEUTIC HYPOTHERMIA IN BRAIN INJURY

Edited by **Farid Sadaka**

Therapeutic Hypothermia in Brain Injury

http://dx.doi.org/10.5772/3380
Edited by Farid Sadaka

Contributors

Rekha Lakshmanan, Farid Sadaka, Ashok Palagiri, Edgar A. Samaniego, David E. Tannehill, Christopher Veremakis, Rahul Nanchal, Gagan Kumar, Kacey B. Anderson, Samuel M. Poloyac

Published by InTech

Janeza Trdine 9, 51000 Rijeka, Croatia

Publishing Process Manager Ana Pantar
Typesetting InTech DTP Team
Cover InTech Design Team

Additional hard copies can be obtained from orders@intechopen.com

Therapeutic Hypothermia in Brain Injury, Edited by Farid Sadaka
p. cm.
ISBN 978-953-51-0960-0

For EU product safety concerns:
IN TECH d.o.o., Prolaz Marije Krucifikse Kozulić 3, 51000 Rijeka, Croatia,
info@intechopen.com or visit our website at intechopen.com.

Meet the editor

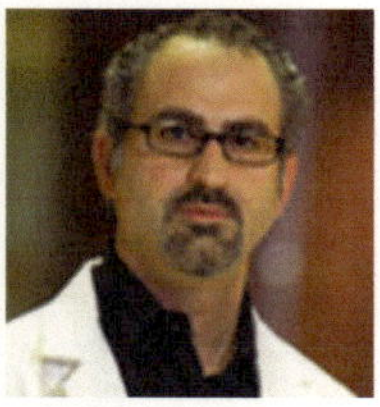

Farid Sadaka is certified by the American Board of Internal Medicine in Internal Medicine and Critical Care Medicine and by the United Council of Neurologic Subspecialties in Neurocritical care. Dr Sadaka is the medical director of the Neurologic and Trauma ICU at Mercy Hospital St Louis, and is also on teaching faculty at St Louis University. Dr Sadaka is an active member of the Society of Critical Care Medicine and Neurocritical Care Society. Dr Sadaka has been invited to speak at several academic centers nationally and locally, on topics pertaining to sepsis and the microcirculation and Therapeutic Hypothermia. Dr Sadaka is actively involved in clinical research. He has had several peer-reviewed publications and book chapters, especially pertaining to neuroscience, traumatic brain injury, sepsis and the microcirculation.

Contents

Preface

This book is meant to look at the evidence behind the application of Therapeutic Hypothermia on patients with injury to the Central Nervous System, including both brain and spinal cord. Central nervous system injury includes ischemia reperfusion after cardiac arrest or asphyxiation, traumatic brain injury, acute ischemic stroke, hemorrhagic stroke, refractory intracranial hypertension, cerebral edema in acute liver failure, subarachnoid hemorrhage, as well as spinal cord injury (SCI). In the minutes to hours following injury, cascades of destructive events and pathophysiologic processes begin at the cellular level. These result in further neuronal injury and are termed the secondary injury. Cellular mechanisms of secondary injury include all of the following: apoptosis, mitochondrial dysfunction, excitotoxicity, disruption in ATP metabolism, disruption in calcium homeostasis, increase in inflammatory mediators and cells, free radical formation, DNA damage, blood-brain barrier disruption, brain glucose utilization disruption, microcirculatory dysfunction and microvascular thrombosis. All of these processes in the brain and spinal cord are temperature dependent; they are all stimulated by fever, and can all be mitigated or blocked by mild to moderate hypothermia. As a result, there has recently been extensive interest in studying the application of Therapeutic Hypothermia (TH) to brain and spinal cord injured patients. This book will discuss the mechanisms by which therapeutic hypothermia can mitigate the pathophysiologies responsible for secondary brain injury, as well as the available evidence for the use of therapeutic hypothermia in multiple neurologic injuries (stated above). Recent studies have indicated that TH with a reduction of body core temperature (T) to 32 - 34 °C for 12 to 24 hours has improved survival and neurologic outcome in comatose out-of-hospital cardiac arrest patients. In this patient population, the evidence for TH is overwhelming leading to major international associations giving it a class I recommendation. However, the evidence for its application to patients with other forms of brain injury stated above and SCI is less overwhelming and still in progress. This book will describe the clinical human evidence behind therapeutic hypothermia for all of the above mentioned brain and spinal cord injuries, as well as the basic and animal studies that led to its clinical applications. This book will also describe how to apply hypothermia to patients with brain injury in the intensive care unit (ICU), methods of cooling and technologies used to induce and maintain therapeutic hypothermia, protocol development for hospitals and ICUs, as well as timing, depth, duration, and management of side-effects.

Neuroprognostication of patients with brain injury and SCI is also significantly affected by the application of therapeutic hypothermia. This book will also describe how hypothermia can influence the ability to prognosticate these injured patients, as well as describe the current evidence to help clinicians offer the family the best and most honest discussion on prognosis of their loved ones. We will also describe how TH influences the metabolism of the most commonly used drugs in the ICU, and how this effect is also linked to prognostication of these patients with brain and spinal cord injury. It will also provide grounds for future directions in the application of and research with therapeutic hypothermia.

Farid Sadaka, MD
Clinical Associate Professor
Critical Care Medicine/ NeuroCritical Care
Medical Director, Trauma and Neuro ICU
Mercy Hospital St Louis/ St. Louis University
St. Louis,
USA

Section 1

Therapeutic Hypothermia-General

Chapter 1

Therapeutic Hypothermia: Adverse Events, Recognition, Prevention and Treatment Strategies

Rekha Lakshmanan, Farid Sadaka and Ashok Palagiri

Additional information is available at the end of the chapter

http://dx.doi.org/10.5772/55022

1. Introduction

Therapeutic hypothermia has been around for centuries, ancient Egyptians, Greeks, and Romans have used it.

Hypothermia is any body temperature below 36 degree C.

Therapeutic Hypothermia is induced hypothermia and can be mild (34-35.9 degree C), moderate (32-33.9 degree C), moderately deep (30.1-31.9 degree C) or deep (less than 30degree C).

Cardiopulmonary resuscitation	Class-I
Traumatic brain injury (ICP CONTROL)	Class I
Traumatic brain injury (outcome)	Class IIa
Stroke	Class-III
Fever in patients with neurological injury	Class IIb
Subarachnoid hemorrhage- vasospasm prevention	Class-IV
Intraoperative hypothermia for intracerebral aneurysm surgery	Class-IIb
Intraoperative hypothermia for thoraco-abdominal aortic aneurysm	Class-III

Figure 1. Current indications for induced therapeutic hypothermia

2. Cardiac arrest

Despite advances in ICU care, cardiac arrest remains a significant cause of death in many countries. Mortality reports vary from 65 to 95% for out-of hospital cardiac arrest. I is a class –I recommendation now that after return of spontaneous circulation in out-of-hospital VF cardiac arrest , patients that remain comatose should be subjected to hypothermia at 32°C to 34°C for 12 to 24 hours. This may also be applied to comatose adult patients with spontaneous circulation after OHCA from a non VF rhythm or in-hospital cardiac arrest.[1]

Several unanswered questions however remain, due to lack of randomized studies. These in part, relate to time from initiation of therapy to achieving target temperature, and whether this is a significant predictor of outcome. The optimal rate of cooling is also an unanswered question, so is the optimal duration of TH in some settings, albeit in the setting of cardiac arrest, improved outcomes have been demonstrated with 12 and 24 hrs of TH at 32°C to 34°C. Hypothermia for neonatal asphyxia is commonly performed for 72 hrs, while hypothermia for cerebral edema associated with liver failure has been reported for as long as 5 days. [2]

3. TBI

Traumatic brain injury (TBI) is a leading cause of death and disability in young people in Western countries. The neuroprotectant effects are thought to be related to decreased metabolic rate, cerebral blood flow, decreased release of excitatory neurotransmitters, decreased apoptosis, cerebral edema, decreased cytokine response etc.[3]

While studies have shown that Hypothermia is clearly effective in controlling intracranial hypertension (level of evidence: class I); it has been difficult to show that lowering ICP definitely improves outcomes. Few positive studies with regard to survival and improved neurological outcome have been shown mainly in tertiary referral centers with experience in use of hypothermia. Here again, as in cardiac arrest, more unanswered questions remain- duration, time of cooling and rewarming, type of rewarming. Currently, most centers perform it for at least 48 hours. Rewarming is typically done slowly, over at least 24 h (level of evidence: class IIa). [4] If there is evidence of ICP elevation during rewarming, again no definite recommendations are available, but most experts will proceed with repeat cooling. It could be that in traumatic brain injury, other therapies, including cerebrospinal fluid drainage, osmolar therapies, sedation, barbiturate coma, and decompressive craniectomy may confer additional benefits that may make it more difficult to prove that Therapeutic hypothermia is superior.

4. Stroke

Similar to Cardiac arrest and TBI there is evidence from animal studies that show benefits of therapeutic hypothermia in stroke. Use of hypothermia in stroke remains experimental, until large prospective randomized human clinical trials using hypothermia in acute stroke are completed. [5]

5. MI

Hypothermia may decrease infarct size in patients with acute myocardial infarction after emergency percutaneous coronary intervention

6. Other indications

Intraoperative hypothermia is used during neurological surgery but without strong evidence from randomized controlled trials. Indications are being studied in the areas of SAH, Neurosurgery, liver failure, Spinal cord injury.

7. Induction of hypothermia

Methods [6]

Both Invasive and non invasive cooling methods have been developed and used to induce hypothermia. The ideal cooling technique should offer efficacy, speed of cooling for target organs, and offer ease of use and transport. It should also have the ability to provide controlled rewarming.

Surface cooling: [Dine et al]

Surface cooling as a noninvasive method to induce hypothermia is easy to use, on the other hand requires more time to achieve the target temperature. There are two described methods: generalized cooling, and selective brain cooling.

Generalized cooling is achieved through the use of cooling blankets, ice packs, and cooling pads. Care should be paid to prevent cold injury to the patient's skin. This method has variability in time to cooling, ranging from 0.03 to 0.98 °C per hour and difficulty in titration of temperature.

Pads that provide direct thermal conduction through the skin are also used; these are unlike conventional water blankets or wraps where heat transfer is by convection. The cooling rate is reported to be 1.5°C/hour or more. Hydrogel-coated pads in these circulate temperature-controlled water under negative pressure, and are placed usually on the patient's abdomen, back and thighs.

Selective brain cooling is another non invasive method. The most commonly used methods are cooling caps and helmets that contain a solution of aqueous glycerol to facilitate heat exchange. Helmet devices do not appear to provide particularly significant protection to the brain, but they reduce core temperature slowly.

Several other limitations exist in surface cooling methods. Through vasoconstriction, shivering, redirection of blood flow away from extremities, they create thermal energy. Overcooling occurs. In a study involving 32 patients where surface cooling was used to induce hypothermia, 63% of patients were overcooled, increasing the risk for adverse events. Another problem with surface cooling is cold injury, causing pressure ulcers and skin breakdown. Surface cooling is less efficient in reducing the temperature of target organs, such as the brain and heart[6]

Invasive cooling

30 ml/kg Lactated Ringers solution that has been chilled to 4°C can be infused over 30 minutes. No adverse effects of the rapid infusion of this volume of IV crystalloid fluid in a study by Bernard. This is followed by another method to maintain hypothermia. Different types of fluids can be used, including 0.9% sodium chloride injection, lactated Ringer's injection, and albumin. Studies have reported cooling rates of 0.8–1.2 °C per liter of fluid infused. Some experts caution that in patients unable to handle the fluid challenge, infusion of large volumes of intravenous fluids in the presence of pulmonary edema or chronic renal failure requiring dialysis may increase adverse events. However , several studies have shown that this process has not been associated with worsening pulmonary edema.[7]

Endovascular cooling is another invasive method used. This is achieved by inserting central venous catheters, with an external heat exchange-control device that circulates cold intravenous fluid. The user sets a target temperature, and the device appropriately adjusts the fluid /water temperature. These devices can reduce temperatures at rates close to 4 °C per hour. In a study by Holzer and colleagues, looking at post cardiac arrest patients, endovascular cooling was found to improve survival and short-term neurologic recovery without higher rates of adverse events, compared with standard treatment. Furthermore, the constant rate of rewarming prevents elevations in ICP. As with any central venous catheters, insertion risks and infectious, bleeding complications may occur. The placement of catheters with associated risks and, and costs of placing them need to be factored. [8]

Other methods for invasive cooling that are reported include cold carotid infusions, single carotid artery perfusion with extracorporeal cooled blood, ice water nasal lavage, cold peritoneal and lung lavage and nasogastric and rectal lavage

Monitoring temperature

Temperature must be monitored continuously and accurately during TH. Peripheral and core temperatures may not always correlate, so two methods of monitoring are usually recommended. A true core temperature is obtained from a pulmonary artery catheter. Tympanic temperatures poorly reflect core temperature. Bladder temperatures are easily obtained by temperature-sensing indwelling urinary catheters. Studies have shown that bladder temperatures are continuous, safe and reliable, correlate well with fluctuations in core temperature. Clinicians must be mindful that in oliguric patients, bladder temperature may poorly reflect core temperature, and other monitoring sites should be used. There is also a delay in reflecting core temperature changes, before bladder temperature also changes, especially the more rapid the cooling rate. This is more of a problem with rectal temperatures. Education of the caregivers about this helps prevent undercooling or overcooling the patient, thereby helps to mitigate the risk of adverse events. [Stone, Gilbert J et al]

8. Phases of temperature modulation in therapeutic hypothermia[2]

Temperature modulation during therapeutic hypothermia may be broken down into four phases: induction, maintenance, rewarming/ decooling, and normothermia. Each of these phases requires monitoring for and prevention of associated complications.(please refer to Figure 2 for an example of a therapeutic hypothermia protocol used in our institution for cardiac arrest patients).

DO NOT SUBSTITUTE **STAT MEDICATION ORDER**

PLEASE INCLUDE: PHYSICIAN NAME, NUMBER AND SIGNATURE

✓	DATE	TIME	**Hypothermia Induction Order Set** **Page 1 of 2**
			Indication: **Patient weight:** **kg**
			☒ NS - 30 mL/kg IV of cold injection at a target of 4° Celsius **STAT**
			☒ Initiate cooling with the appropriate hypothermia induction device according to Hypothermia Induction policy
			☒ Apply pads appropriate for patient weight(Apply Universal pads if Wt>= 220 LBs)
			☒ The Arctic Sun is preset to 33° Celsius
			☒ Start Magnesium Sulphate 4 Gm IV (in 100 ml injectable water) over 4 hours
			Nursing
			☒ Continuous cardiac monitoring with pulse oximetry - monitor vital signs and record every hour
			☒ Consider target MAP ≥ 90mmHg or mmHg to maintain Cerebral Perfusion Pressure (CPP) of ___
			☒ Goal CVP 8-12mmHg or mmHg ☒ Maintain ScvO2 > 70%.(if available)
			☒ Obtain bedside glucose every 1 hour. (See Adult Insulin order sheet if already initiated.)Maintain Accuchecks q 1 Hr until T=37° Celsius.(maintain BS=110-150)
			☒ ABG every hour(s)
			☒ CBC, BMP, Magnesium, Phosphorus, PT/PTT every 6 hours
			☒ Consider blood cultures 12 hours after initiation of cooling
			☒ Initiate VAP Bundle Order Set, if not already begun
			☒ No sedation vacation if patient is receiving neuromuscular blockade infusion or in cooling phase
			☒ Consider Empiric Antimicrobial therapy if sepsis or immunosuppression is suspected(ex: neutropenia..)
			Activity
			☒ Bedrest
			☒ Skin assessment should be performed and documented every 4 hours
			☒ Turn patient every two hours unless contraindicated and ordered
			☒ PT/OT consults and treatment if not already ordered
			Sedation/Analgesia/Control of Shivering
			☒ Propofol (DIPRIVAN) drip initiated at 10mcg/kg/min. - titrate by 5mcg/kg/min for Ramsay of ____ to a max. of 80mcg/kg/min
			☒ Midazolam (VERSED) drip initiated at mg/hour - titrate by 1mg/hr for Ramsay of ____
			☒ Fentanyl infusion at mcg/hour - titrate to mcg/hour
			☒ Morphine infusion at mg/hour - titrate to mg/hour
			If still shivering (physical assessment or trend indicator) give:
			☒Buspar 10mg/ 20mg PT TID(circle dose)
✓	DATE	TIME	**Hypothermia Induction Order Set** **Page 2 of 2**
			If still shivering, consider neuromuscular blockade:
			☒ Start with PRN dosing as ordered for shivering ☒ If patient still shivering, consider continuous infusion. ☒ Place "Neuromuscular Blockade in use" sign at head of bed.
			☒ Atracurium ☒ Intermittent dosing____________(dose/route/interval) ☒ Loading dose (0.5 mg/kg) = _______ mg IV x one dose now ☒ Infusion – begin at 4 mcg/kg/min IV to a max. of 12 mcg/kg/min
			☒ Vecuronium ☒ Intermittent dosing____________(dose/route/interval) ☒ Loading dose (0.1 mg/kg) = _______ mg IV x one dose now ☒ Infusion – begin at 1 mcg/kg/min IV to a max. of 2 mcg/kg/min

			Paralytic Titration
			☒ Monitor patient for ventilator compliance and shivering
			Continuous EEG(please choose one of the following):
			☒ Start now and D/C when patient is rewarmed to 37° Celsius - page EEG tech
			☒ Start in am and D/C when patient is rewarmed to 37° Celsius - page EEG tech
			Respiratory: ☒ Maintain O2 Sats=95% ☒ Maintain pCO2=40mmHg
			Medications
			☒ Artificial tears ophthalmic ointment (LACRILUBE or equivalent) – one ribbon in each eye every 12 hours.
			☒ Maintenance IV Fluids: at ml/hr.-**Titrate to maintain equal to UO.**
			Rewarming - To start 24 hours after temperature of 33° Celsius is attained
			☒ Continuous EKG for dysrhythmias
			☒ Stop all potassium infusions
			☒ Rewarm at 0.25° Celsius to 0.33° Celsius per hour - ☒ Keep patient in goal temperature range of 36° Celsius to 37° Celsius for next 48 hours
			☒ May discontinue paralytic(if used) once goal temperature is obtained
			☒ Begin daily sedation vacation once paralytic has been discontinued
			Once rewarmed, please maintain EUTHERMIA(~37° Celsius).

Figure 2. Mercy Hospital St Louis In-HOSPITAL Therapeutic Hypothermia Protocol

In the setting of cardiac arrest, based on animal and human data, initiation of cooling should be done as soon as possible after return of spontaneous circulation (ROSC). The induction phase can be initiated in the prehospital or in hospital setting. There are ongoing studies involving prehospital cooling. One should be mindful that if prehospital cooling is not followed by in hospital cooing, outcomes could be considerably worse, especially if patients are rewarmed quickly

The maintenance phase usually occurs in an intensive care unit and hemodynamic parameters, electrolytes should be watched closely. For example, hypokalemia is a common occurrence, and can precipitate further arrests, so replacement is essential. Secondary insults such as hypercarbia, hypoxemia, glycemic shifts should be avoided. It is important to recognize that drug metabolism is altered in hypothermia, meticulous attention to medication dosing is needed and aggressive treatment of shivering, with sedation and neuromuscular blockade is often needed

Fever in the first 72 hrs after ROSC is associated with poor outcome. Although unproven, an increasing body of evidence supports the cautious prevention and treatment of fever in the setting of critical neurological illness, and many clinicians attempt to maintain a core temperature of 36°C to 37.5°C until at least 72 hrs after ROSC

Rewarming /Decooling is associated with electrolyte shifts, vasodilation, and the "post resuscitation" syndrome, many deaths occur in this phase due to hemodynamic instability and other complications. Rewarming / Decooling should not be treated casually.

The "post resuscitation" syndrome which is characterized by elevated inflammatory cytokine levels, vasodilatory shock, intracranial hypertension, and thereby decreased cerebral perfusion pressure often compounds the myocardial dysfunction related to acute myocardial infarction, defibrillation injury or cardiomyopathy. The duration of cooling and rewarming may vary depending on the indication, for instance, in post cardiac arrest, rewarming is usually begun 24 hours after the initiation of cooling, in intracranial hypertension, this is typically done later, after 48 hours. Patients should be rewarmed slowly so that it avoids rapid hemodynamic alterations, while preserving the neuroprotectant effects of hypothermia. The usual rate of rewarming is a goal rate of 0.2°C to 0.33°C per hour, in ICP elevations; the rate is sometimes slower, at 0.05 to 0.1 degrees C per hour. While the optimal rewarming rate remains unknown; the process usually takes about 8 hours. Careful hemodynamic monitoring is needed, patients may require additional hemodynamic support with fluid boluses, inotropes, and vasopressors to maintain adequate cerebral perfusion pressures, and mean arterial pressures during decooling, Sometimes, if significant hemodynamic instability or signs of elevated ICP occur, it may become necessary to slow or stop the temperature decooling process. Rewarming is typically achieved through active or passive means through the use of heated-air blankets, or the removal of cooling methods allowing the patient's body temperature to increase over time. Paralysis and sedation should be maintained until the patient's temperature reaches 35 °C. Patients must be monitored closely, and all electrolyte infusions must be discontinued to avoid dangerous electrolyte shifts

Physiological effects of hypothermia

Hypothermia affects many intracellular processes. While some of these are directly related to its protective effects, hypothermia therapy is also known to be associated with a number of potential adverse events. These adverse effects generally do not pose a problem until core body temperatures are< 35°C.

Many physiological, laboratory changes occur with induction of hypothermia. Education of caregivers is key, so there is not only timely recognition of adverse events, but unnecessary interventions are minimized in case of routine changes that are seen. It is possible that in many studies especially in traumatic brain injury and hypothermia, the results may have been negatively impacted by adverse events related to hypothermia and /or failure to recognize and treat the physiological effects.

Example, mild hypothermia is associated leucopenia, thrombocytopenia. Hyperglycemia is common due to decreased insulin sensitivity and increased insulin resistance. Decreases in cardiac output may be seen, also an increase in lactate levels and levels of serum transaminases, amylase. A common occurrence is increased urinary output (cold diuresis). These effects of hypothermia depend on the degree of hypothermia, age, comorbidities. A significant risk for severe arrhythmias occurs at temperatures below 28–30°C. These low temperatures are not typically used in current practice; the target temperature is usually mild –moderate hypothermia, although they are still practiced in major vascular and other neurosurgical procedures.[4]

Hypothermia leads to a decrease in the metabolic rate. Metabolism is reduced by between 5% and 7% per Celsius degree reduction in body temperature. Cerebral blood flow is decreased, but, this is offset by the decrease in metabolism. It decreases cerebral edema, decreases the excessive influx of Ca2+ into the cell, decreases the accumulation of glutamate, an excitatory neurotransmitter. It thereby is thought to decrease apoptosis.

Hypothermia inhibits neutrophil and macrophage function, suppresses inflammatory reactions and inhibits the release of pro-inflammatory cytokines. While this may help contribute to hypothermia's neuroprotective effects, this may occur at the expense of an increased the risk of infections.

Shivering	Increased muscle activity, increased oxygen consumption, increased rate of metabolism
Drug metabolism	Altered clearance of various medications
Cardiovascular EKG **Manifestations**	prolonged P-R and Q-T intervals and widening of the QRS
Arrhythmias	tachycardia, and then bradycardia, atrial fibrillation
Infection	inhibits the release of various pro-inflammatory cytokines, inhibit neutrophil and macrophage function
Coagulopathy	increased bleeding time, increased APTT/CT, thrombocytopenia
Electrolyte disorders	Hypokalemia, Hypomagnesemia during cooling, hyperkalemia during rewarming
Insulin resistance	hyperglycemia

Figure 3. Adverse events of Hypothermia, prevention and management strategies:

Shivering

Shivering is the body's physiological response to hypothermia. Both in the induction and maintenance of hypothermia, this can pose challenges, and shivering is sometimes more an issue when normothermia is the goal temperature. Shivering generates heat and increases the oxygen consumption and metabolic demands of tissues.

Shivering is especially important in the extremes of age. It has been associated with a higher risk of adverse cardiac events and poor outcomes in the perioperative setting. The threshold for shivering is slightly higher in females. The process is regulated via the preoptic nucleus of the anterior hypothalamus. Through positive and negative feedback loops this helps minimize fluctuations, maintains core body temperature within 0.1°C– 0.2°C. [4]

Typically a shivering response is seen when core temperature decreases below 35.5°C, the "shivering threshold." However, in febrile patients, and in brain injured patients, this regulation is altered and both the temperature "set point" and the shivering threshold increase. The hypothalamus then makes attempts to maintain the higher temperatures as it does to maintain normal temperature or normothermia. This causes an increase in oxygen consumption, metabolic rate, and increases carbon dioxide production. At temperatures lower than 33-34°C, the shivering response decreases, therefore sedation and paralytics can be decreased at this point, if the clinical situation allows it.

The Bedside Shivering Assessment Scale (BSAS) is a simple scale that was developed as a means to detect and quantify shivering and guide therapeutic interventions. The scale has 4 levels. [9]

Score	Description or observation	Severity
0	Absence of shivering on palpation of neck or pectoralis muscles	None
1	Localized to the neck and/or thorax	Mild
2	Involvement of the upper extremities with or without neck	Moderate
3	Generalized, whole-body involvement	Severe

Table 1. Bedside Shivering assessment Scale

A non pharmacologic measure that has been shown to decrease shivering in some studies, mainly in healthy volunteers is called Surface counter warming. Studies have shown decreased shivering and improved metabolic profiles, and that is safe and effective, easy to use. Theoretically, an increase of 4°C in skin temperature could compensate for a 1°C decrease in core temperature, reducing the shivering response.[9]

Numerous pharmacologic strategies have been used to control shivering. In the operating room, volatile anesthetics, including halothane, isoflurane and enflurane, are used to control post anesthetic shivering. In the intensive care unit, other agents are of more practical use. These agents are thought to be effective by various mechanisms. The agents act though serotonin manipulation, or are N-methyl-D-aspartate Antagonists, α_2-agonists, Opioids, and others. Most studies involving these agents have been conducted in healthy volunteers.

Buspirone is a serotonin (5-HT) 1A partial agonist that has been shown to be a good anti shivering agent. At a 60-mg dose, buspirone – a 5-HT1a partial agonist – reduced the shivering threshold by 0.7°C. A study in volunteers found that a 30-mg dose combined with low-dose meperidine produced a similar reduction in shivering threshold compared to a large dose of meperidine alone (2.3°C).Buspirone provides a good synergistic therapy when combined with other antishivering interventions. The main disadvantage of buspirone is that it needs to be administered enterally, no IV formulation is available. Bioavailability in the critically ill may not be reliable.[10]

Meperidine is an opioid analgesic. Meperidine is probably the single most useful antishivering drug, but has significant adverse events. Meperidine acts on both mu and kappa receptors, is considered the most effective antishivering agent among the opioids. The mechanism behind meperidine's antishivering action is not clearly known. It is thought that activation of [kappa]-opioid receptors, anticholinergic action, and N-methyl-d-aspartate antagonism all play a role. In studies, plasma concentrations near 1.3 μg/mL have been required to induce moderate hypothermia with meperidine alone, which could increase the risk of side effects. Meperidine is effective for postoperative shivering and, it inhibits shivering twice as much as vasoconstriction.

Meperidine has major side effects; the more significant of them is lowering of seizure threshold. Other reported adverse events include arrhythmias, hyperreflexia, and myoclonus. The metabolite Normeperidine accumulates in patients with renal failure and could potentiate these adverse events.

Fentanyl, morphine are pure mu opioid receptor agonists, and have had mixed results in studies. High doses may be needed to achieve this effect, and this may potentiate side effects[11].

The alpha$_2$-receptor agonists are another important class of drugs used as pharmacologic measures to control shivering. Bradycardia and hypotension are the main adverse events with this class of drugs. Important to remember, they may also exacerbate the bradycardia induced by hypothermia.

Clonidine decreases the vasoconstriction and shivering thresholds. Prophylactic use of clonidine lowered the threshold of vasoconstriction in healthy volunteers. [12, 13] In a trial comparing clonidine and meperidine, the average onset of action for meperidine and clonidine were 2.7 and 3.1 minutes, respectively. At least from these data, clonidine appears to be as effective as meperidine for postanesthetic shivering[14]

Dexmedetomidine is another agent that has been shown to decrease postanesthetic shivering when compared to both placebo and Meperidine. In studies with dexmedetomidine in healthy volunteers, it showed a decrease in the vasoconstriction and shivering thresholds by similar amounts.[15]

A small study looked at healthy volunteers and found that Meperidine and Dexmedetomidine were synergistic as well. [16, 17]

Magnesium is another anti shivering agent. It is thought to act as an antagonist of the NMDA receptors. In addition, hypothermia causes hypomagnesaemia commonly, and magnesium replacement is often required. Results on magnesium as a neuroprotectant have been variable. In a study of healthy volunteers, despite reducing the shivering threshold, the authors concluded that it was not clinically significant in counteracting the shivering effect of therapeutic hypothermia. [18] In another study, magnesium shortened the time to achieve target temperature and improved patient comfort.

In this small study, 22 volunteers were randomly assigned to one of four therapies: meperidine monotherapy; meperidine plus buspirone; meperidine plus ondansetron; or meperidine, ondansetron, and magnesium sulfate. In this study, Magnesium was shown to decrease time to target temperature and increase patient comfort. Although the presence of shivering was recorded in this investigation, these data were not reported. [19]

Dantrolene is another agent that has been used for malignant hyperthermia. It acts on the skeletal muscle and interferes with the release of calcium from the sarcoplasmic reticulum, and inhibits the excitation-contraction coupling of skeletal muscles. It is a good adjunctive antishivering agent. In a study with healthy volunteers, dantrolene decreased the gain of shivering. Dantrolene had no effect on the vasoconstriction threshold. Hepatitis is a complication of dantrolene, especially in people older than 35 years. The reaction can be dose dependent or idiosyncratic.[20]

Propofol has been widely studied in Shivering control. It has been compared to Thiopental and isoflurane. Patients on propofol experienced less shivering compared to thiopental alone or thiopental plus isoflurane. Like other drugs, during hypothermia, the plasma concentration of propofol is increased by 30% due to reduced clearance. Clinicians should also be aware of propofol infusion syndrome.[21] [22] Propofol infusion syndrome is a rare complication of propofol infusion. Risk factors include administration of high doses (greater than 3-5 mg/kg per) and prolonged use, more than 48 hours, patients on catecholamines for vasopressor support, steroids. Additional proposed risk factors include a young age, critical illness, high fat and low carbohydrate intake, inborn errors of mitochondrial fatty acid oxidation. Patients present with cardiac dysrhythmias, metabolic acidosis, rhabdomyolysis, and renal failure. It can be associated with a high mortality.

There is limited data on the use of other agents such as Ketamine, methylphenidate and doxapram as anti shivering agents in hypothermia.

Drug metabolism

By redistributing blood flow away from muscle, skin, and fat, hypothermia alters drug pharmacokinetics. Drugs with a large volume of distribution, in the setting of hypothermia distribute to reduced volume and thereby produce higher plasma concentrations. Due to reduced blood flow, these drugs may initially be sequestered in tissue, but subsequently with rewarming and vasodilation, these drugs now redistribute from tissues, leading to high plasma concentrations, thereby increasing the risk of toxicity.[23]

Cardiovascular manifestations

Cardiac output decreases, but this is offset by the decreased metabolic rate

Common electrocardiographic findings during hypothermia include prolonged P-R and Q-T intervals and widening of the QRS complex as well as altered T waves and appearance of the J wave. (Osborne). These usually do not require interventions.

Arrhythmias: Initially, hypothermia causes tachycardia, and then bradycardia ensues. The arrhythmias depend on the severity of hypothermia, more severe commonly occur at temperatures of < 28C. The bradycardia may be severe enough to warrant discontinuing hypothermia. This is compounded by the fact that the anti arrhythmics become less effective, and so does electrical defibrillation. Attempts at electrical defibrillation can initiate malignant arrhythmias.

In the setting of a cardiac arrest, the myocardium in a deeply hypothermic patient is easily susceptible to manipulations such as CPR, defibrillation, and can predispose to arrhythmias.

While mild hypothermia can be protective by stabilizing membranes, severe hypothermia increases risk of malignant arrhythmias.

Limited data exist on the efficacy of various antiarrhythmics. Bretylium, the most commonly studied agent, has been recommended as the drug of choice during moderate-to-severe hypothermia

Observational data from humans and experimental animal models have looked at Bretylium. Bretylium is a parenteral Class III antiarrhythmic agent. However, Bretylium is no longer available in the US secondary to lack of availability of raw materials needed to produce the drug, as well as declining usage in clinical practice. Amiodarone has been studied in an animal model. Stoner et al looked at thirty anesthetized dogs and induced hypothermic VF. They compared defibrillation rates after drug therapy with amiodarone, bretylium, and placebo. In this study, neither amiodarone nor bretylium was significantly better than placebo in improving the resuscitation rate.[24, 25.]The benefits of amiodarone during hypothermia have not been clearly established in humans. In the Bernard study looking at hypothermia after cardiac arrest, Lidocaine was administered for 24 hrs. Clinically significant cardiac arrhythmias occurred with less frequency in the Australian study compared to the European study, where no lidocaine was employed. [6]

Coronary blood flow has been shown to decrease during mild hypothermia in patients with coronary artery disease. Evidence from animal studies has shown a 10% reduction in myocardial infarct size for every 1°C decrease in body temperature. [26]

Dixon et al looked at a randomized study of 42 patients with acute myocardial infarction and where cooling was maintained for 3 hours after reperfusion (core temperature target 33 degrees C.)There were no significant adverse hemodynamic events with cooling; however, the median infarct size was not significantly smaller in those that were cooled compared with the control group[27]

Other clinical studies of therapeutic hypothermia in patients with acute myocardial infarction who are undergoing primary PCI have not shown any beneficial effects.

Despite these data, hypothermia can potentially cause hypotension and myocardial dysfunction. It induces a cold diuresis and induces hypovolemia. This is through increased venous return, stimulation of atrial natriuretic peptide, decreased anti diuretic hormone levels, and renal tubular dysfunction.

Patients with severe Traumatic brain injury may also receive mannitol for hyperosmolar therapy for raised intracranial pressures or may have diabetes insipidus, which can further contribute to hypovolemia.[4]

Infection

Infectious complications occur frequently in ICU patients, especially after cardiac arrest. The increasing use of therapeutic hypothermia has raised awareness about increased infectious complications. In a retrospective review of a single institution cohort, Mongardon et al found that pneumonia as the most common source, and Staphylococcus aureus was the main causative agent. Duration of hypothermia was associated with increased infection rates. ICU survival and neurologic outcome were not affected. [28]A numbers of studies, especially in patients with stroke or TBI, have reported higher risks of pneumonia when therapeutic hypothermia is used over longer periods of time (48–72 h) However, other studies using hypothermia for prolonged periods in patients with TBI reported no increase in infection rates.

Evidence from clinical and in vitro studies shows that hypothermia can impair immune function. Hypothermia inhibits the release of various pro-inflammatory cytokines, inhibit neutrophil and macrophage function. Kimura and colleagues found that the peak release of interleukin-6, interleukin-1, and other proinflammatory cytokines was significantly delayed at 33 °C compared with 37 °C [29, 30] Hypothermia reduces gastrointestinal motility, and cardiac dysfunction in post arrest patients, therefore, it may increase risk of mucosal ischemia and breakdown. This may cause bacterial translocation. The insulin resistance and hyperglycemia associated with hypothermia may further predispose the patient to infection. The normal host responses to infection like leukocytosis may not be noted in hypothermic patients, so careful surveillance is needed. The threshold to initiate antibiotic treatment should be low. Fever in these patients should be treated aggressively to prevent further neurologic injury.

Many institutions perform blood cultures and sputum cultures at the time of initiation of hypothermia, and periodic surveillance cultures to detect early bacteremia. In patients developing infections after hypothermia treatment, fever should be treated aggressively, to mitigate new or additional neurological injuries

Seizures

In a retrospective observational study involving neonates, moderate cooling decreased seizures recorded by EEG.[31] Seizures after cardiac arrest and TBI are common; the detection of seizures is an important aspect of a neurointensivist in the care of therapeutic hypothermia patients. Many of these patients are under neuromuscular blockade, and convulsive movements are absent. The incidence of seizures after cardiac arrest is around 24%, with some studies showing a higher incidence than others. Continuous EEG monitoring should be used when available over intermittent EEG, because seizures could be no convulsive as well as convulsive in these patients. The disadvantage of continuous EEG is that is not always available, is expensive, labor intensive, and subject to misinterpretation. No clear guidelines exist to guide therapy of EEG findings like PLEDS.

Intravenous benzodiazepines are used the initial medical treatment of status epilepticus. If the patient fails first line therapy and is considered to be in refractory status epilepticus, there is no firm data to guide subsequent management. The VA cooperative study showed that early control with a first line agent is important, because, if the first line agent fails, the success of subsequent second and third line agents is marginal. In the VA cooperative trial, the treatment success rate with the first drug was 55% in the overt status group and 15% in the subtle status group.[32, 33]

Many experts recommend continuous intravenous antiepileptic drugs at this stage. Midazolam is the safest anesthetic agent in treating SE. Doses as high as 3 to 5 mg/kg/h may be necessary to maintain seizure suppression in the most refractory cases. Tachyphylaxis is often encountered when prolonged infusions are used. The other agents used to treat SE are propofol, and barbiturates (Thiopental or pentobarbital). Barbiturates produce hypotension, and myocardial depression, this may pose further challenges in the post cardiac arrest setting. Other side effects include ileus, hepatotoxicity, increased susceptibility to infections and very prolonged sedation. Propofol can be associated with propofol infusion syndrome as discussed earlier. Valproic acid, levetiracetam, are emerging as alternative agents. Fosphenytoin is an antiepileptic that is often added in these patients. Fosphenytoin is a prodrug of phenytoin and its preparation does not include propylene glycol. It can be administered faster than IV phenytoin, and has less adverse cardiac events with IV infusion compared to phenytoin. It is much less likely to produce local tissue reactions, and it can be infused faster than phenytoin.[34] As with status epilepticus from other causes, it is not clear whether burst suppression on EEG is superior to seizure suppression. No data on seizure prophylaxis after hypoxic ischemic encephalopathy are available

9. Coagulation

Bleeding diatheses occur in the setting of mild therapeutic hypothermia. For every 1 °C decrease in temperature, coagulation-factor function is decreased by 10%. Watts et al showed that in trauma patients, enzyme activity alteration, platelet dysfunction and changes in fibrin pathways occur. Clinically significant bleeding is rarely a significant problem, even in traumatic brain injury patients. Schefold et al. in a prospective observational study of 31 patients with AMI and mild induced hypothermia and primary PCI found no excessive bleeding risk with cooling/PCI.[35,36]

Values of standard coagulation tests such as prothrombin time and partial thromboplastin times are usually normal, because these tests are usually performed at 37°C in the lab. Tests will be prolonged only if they are performed at the patient's actual core temperature

10. Pressure ulcers

Skin integrity should be assessed carefully and frequently. The surface cooling, vasoconstrictive response to cooling can increase skin breakdown in hypothermic patients.[6]

11. Gastrointestinal dysfunction

Hypothermia patients have GI dysmotility, ileus. Caution needs to be exercised with promotility agents like Erythromycin, metoclopramide, neostigmine, as they can induce arrhythmias. Increased serum amylase levels are common, but patients rarely have significant pancreatitis. Enteral nutrition can help decrease risk of bacterial translocation. Gaussorgues P, et al. Bacteremia following cardiac arrest and cardiopulmonary resuscitation. *Intensive Care Med* 1988; 14(5):575-7.

12. Hypovolemia, fluid balance and electrolytes, glycemia

A common problem is severe electrolyte disorders hypokalemia, hypomagnesemia, hypophosphatemia during induction of cooling. These may cause further arrhythmias in post-arrest patients. Hypothermia decreases insulin sensitivity and insulin secretion, which often leads to hyperglycemia. Tight control of glucose levels may decrease morbidity and mortality in ICU patients, but the exact levels at which glycemia needs to be maintained is controversial. During rewarming, glucose levels tend to drop, and therefore, insulin may need to be decreased or discontinued. Likewise, hyperkalemia and hypermagnesemia are common during rewarming, and cardiac arrests have occurred when the clinician s unaware of this phenomenon. Hypothermia also induces a metabolic acidosis by increased synthesis of glycerol, free fatty acids, ketones and lactate. These changes are normal metabolic consequences of hypothermia and should not be attributed to complications such as bowel ischemia.[4]

Hypotension can occur through hypovolemia, the cold diuresis, that occurs in hypothermia, and the use of agents like mannitol in TBI or diuretics in the setting of cardiomyopathies can further exacerbate this. If this is unrecognized, the problem is worse in the rewarming phase when vasodilatation often occurs, and profound shock ensues. [Cueni-Villoz N, et al.]

13. Summary

In conclusion, hypothermia is becoming increasingly used across many intensive care units, and the applications could expand well beyond the current indications. It is important to use safe, effective cooling methods, recognize, prevent and treat various adverse events that could occur, so we can improve the survival of these patients.

Author details

Rekha Lakshmanan, Farid Sadaka and Ashok Palagiri
Mercy Hospital St. Louis, Missouri, USA

14. References

[1] Nolan JP, Neumar RW, Adrie C, et al. Post-cardiac arrest syndrome: epidemiology, pathophysiology, treatment, and prognostication. A Scientific Statement from the International Liaison Committee on Resuscitation; the American Heart Association Emergency Cardiovascular Care Committee; the Council on Cardiovascular Surgery and Anesthesia; the Council on Cardiopulmonary, Perioperative, and Critical Care; the Council on Clinical Cardiology; the Council on Stroke. Resuscitation 2008;79:350–379

[2] Seder, David B. MD; Van der Kloot, Thomas E. MD Methods of cooling: Practical aspects of therapeutic temperature management. Critical Care Medicine Issue: Volume 37(7) Supplement, July 2009, pp S211-S222

[3] Sosin DM, Sniezek JE, Thurman DJ (1996) Incidence of mild and moderate brain injury in the United States 1991.Brain Injury 10:47–54
[4] Kees H. Polderman Mechanisms of action, physiological effects, and complications of hypothermia Intensive Care Med (2004) 30:757–769
[5] Reith J, Jorgensen HS, Pedersen PM, Nakayama H, Raaschou HO, Jeppesen LL, et al. Body temperature in acute stroke: relation to stroke severity, infarct size, mortality, and outcome. Lancet. Feb 17 1996;347(8999):422-5
[6] LEE, ROZALYNNE; ASARE, KWAME Therapeutic hypothermia for out-of-hospital cardiac arrest American Journal of Health-System Pharmacy Issue: Volume 67(15), 1 August 2010, p 1229–1237
[7] Bernard, S. et al. Induced hypothermia using large volume, ice-cold intravenous fluid in comatose survivors of out-of-hospital cardiac arrest: A preliminary report. Resuscitation 2003;56:9-13
[8] Soga, T. et al. Mild therapeutic hypothermia using extracorporeal cooling method in comatose survivors after out-of-hospital cardiac arrest. Circulation 2006;114:II-1190
[9] Badjatia N, Strongilis E, Gordon E, et al. Metabolic impact of shivering during therapeutic modulation: the Bedside Shivering Assessment Scale. Stroke. 2008;39:3242–3247
[10] Mokhtarani M, et al. Buspirone and meperidine synergistically reduce the shivering threshold. Anesth Analg. 2001; 93(5):1233-9.
[11] Kurz A, et al. Meperidine decreases the shivering threshold twice as much as the vasoconstriction threshold. Anesthesiology. 1997;86(5):1046
[12] Delaunay L, et al. Clonidine comparably decreases the thermoregulatory thresholds for vasoconstriction and shivering in humans. Anesthesiology. 1993;79(3):470
[13] Nicolaou G, et al. Clonidine decreases vasoconstriction and shivering thresholds, without affecting the sweating threshold. Can J Anaesth. 1997;44(6):636
[14] Schwarzkopf KR, et al. A comparison between meperidine, clonidine and urapidil in the treatment of postanesthetic shivering. Anaesth Intensive Care. 2001;92(1):257
[15] Bicer C, et al. Dexmedetomidine and meperidine prevent postanesthetic shivering. Eur J Anaesthesiol. 2006;23(2):149
[16] Doufas AG, Lin CM, Suleman MI, et al. Dexmedetomidine and meperidine additively reduce the shivering threshold in humans. Stroke. 2003; 34:1218–1223.
[17] Talke P, Tayefeh F, Sessler DI, Jeffrey R, Noursalehi M, Richardson C. Dexmedetomidine does not alter the sweating threshold, but comparably and linearly reduces the vasoconstriction and shivering thresholds. Anesthesiology. 1997; 87: 835–841
[18] Anupama Wadhwa, Magnesium Sulfate Only Slightly Reduces the ShiveringThreshold in Humans Br J Anaesth. 2005 June; 94(6): 756–762
[19] Zweifler RM, Voorhees ME, Mahmood MA, Parnell M. Magnesium sulfate increases the rate of hypothermia via surface cooling and improves comfort. Stroke 2004; 35:2331–4.
[20] Lin CM, Neeru S, Doufas AG, et al. Dantrolene reduces the threshold and gain for shivering. Anesth Analg 2004;98:1318–24

[21] Matsukawa T, et al. Propofol linearly reduces the vasoconstriction and shivering thresholds. Anesthesiology. 1995;82(5):1169
[22] Cheong KF, Chen FG, Yau GH. Postanaesthetic shivering--a comparison of thiopentone and propofol. Ann Acad Med Singapore. 1998;27(5):729
[23] Leslie K, Sessler DI, Bjorksten AR, Moayeri A. Mild hypothermia alters propofol pharmacokinetics and increases the duration of action of atracurium. Anesth Analg 1995;80: 1007–14
[24] Stoner J, Martin G, O'Mara K, et al. Amiodarone and bretylium in the treatment of hypothermic ventricular fibrillation in a canine model
[25] Arpino PA and Greer DM. Practical pharmacological aspects of therapeutic hypothermia after cardiac arrest. Pharmacotherapy. 2008; 28:102–11
[26] Chien GL, Wolff RA, Davis RF, Van Winkle DM. "Normothermic range" temperature affects myocardial infarct size. Cardiovasc Res 1994;28:1014-1017
[27] Dixon SR, Whitbourn RJ, Dae MW, et al. Induction of mild systemic hypothermia with endovascular cooling during primary percutaneous coronary intervention for acute myocardial infarction. J Am Coll Cardiol 2002;40:1928–34.
[28] Mongardon, N et al. Infectious complications in out-of-hospital cardiac arrest patients in the therapeutic hypothermia era. Crit Care Med 2011 Vol. 39, No. 6
[29] Kimura A, Sakurada S, Ohkuni H,Todome Y, Kurata K (2002) Moderatehypothermia delays roinflammatory
[30] cytokine production of human peripheralblood mononuclear cells. Crit CareMed 30:1499–1502
[31] Aibiki M, Maekawa S, Ogura S, Kinoshita Y, Kawai N, Yokono S (1999) Effect of moderate hypothermia on systemic and internal jugular plasma IL-6 levels after traumatic brain injury in humans. J Neurotrauma 16:225–232
[32] Low, Evonne; Boylan, Geraldine; Mathieson, Sean R; Murray, Deirdre M; Korotchikova, Irina; Stevenson, Nathan J; Livingstone, Vicki; Rennie, Janet M Cooling and seizure burden in term neonates: an observational study Archives of Disease in Childhood: Fetal and Neonatal Edition Issue: Volume 97(4), July 2012, p F267–F272
[33] Treiman DM, Meyers PD, Walton NY, et al. A comparison of four treatments for generalized convulsive status epilepticus. Veterans affairs status epilepticus cooperative study group. N Engl J Med 1998; 39:792
[34] Meierkord H, Boon P, Engelsen B, et al. EFNS guideline on the management of status epilepticus. Eur J Neurol 2006;13:445–50
[35] Rabinstein AA. Management of Status Epilepticus in Adults Neurol Clin - 01-NOV-2010; 28(4): 53-62
[36] Schefold JC, Storm C, Joerres A, Hasper D. Mild therapeutic hypothermia after cardiac arrest and the risk of bleeding in patients with acute myocardial infarction. International Journal of Cardiology 2009; 132: 387–91
[37] Watts DD, Trask A, Soeken K, et al. Hypothermic coagulopathy in trauma: effect of varying levels of hypothermia on enzyme speed, platelet function, and fibrinolytic activity. J Trauma. 1998; 44:846–54

Additional References:

Therapeutic Hypothermia for Neuroprotection Emerg Med Clin North Am. 2009 Feb;27(1):137-49, ix.C. Jessica Dine, MDa, Benjamin S. Abella, MD, MPhi

Do Standard Monitoring Sites Reflect True Brain Temperature When Profound Hypothermia Is Rapidly Induced and Reversed?. Stone, Gilbert J. MD; Young, William L. MD; Smith, Craig R. MD; Solomon, Robert A. MD; Wald, Alvin PhD; Ostapkovich, Noeleen REPT; Shrebnick, Debra B. PA Anesthesiology. 82(2):344-351, February 1995.

Gaussorgues P, et al. Bacteremia following cardiac arrest and cardiopulmonary resuscitation. *Intensive Care Med* 1988;14(5):575-7.

Cueni-Villoz N, et al. Increased blood glucose variability during therapeutic hypothermia and outcome after cardiac arrest. *Crit Care Med* 2011;39(10):2225-31.

Section 2

Therapeutic Hypothermia-Cardiac Arrest

Chapter 2

Therapeutic Hypothermia for Cardiac Arrest

Farid Sadaka

Additional information is available at the end of the chapter

http://dx.doi.org/10.5772/49374

1. Introduction

In the era before Therapeutic Hypothermia (TH) was recommended and used as a therapeutic modality for out-of-hospital cardiac arrest (OHCA) patients, reported data suggests in-hospital mortality exceeded 58%.[1,2,3,4,5,6] Mortality after a sudden and unexpected cardiac arrest (CA) is high, and the chance of survival to hospital discharge has, until recently, remained unchanged.[7] In one report, OHCA in the U.S. has a mortality rate greater than 90% which results in more than 300,000 deaths per year.[8] Those who survive the devastating event, often retain a hypoxic brain injury and a permanently incapacitating neurologic deficit.[9] Studies of patients who survived to ICU admission but subsequently died in the hospital, brain injury was the cause of death in 68% after out-of-hospital cardiac arrest and in 23% after in-hospital cardiac arrest.[10,11] Therapeutic hypothermia, or targeted temperature management, is a therapeutic intervention that is intended to limit neurologic injury after a patient's resuscitation from cardiac arrest.

2. Mechanisms of neuroprotection

A cascade of destructive events and processes begins at the cellular level in the minutes to hours following an initial injury. These processes, the result of ischemia and reperfusion, may continue for hours to many days after the initial injury.[12] It is crucial to note that all of these processes after ischemic-reperfusion injury in the brain are temperature dependent; they are all stimulated by fever, and can all be mitigated or blocked by hypothermia. Since most of these processes start within minutes to hours after the injury, then application of hypothermia earlier might be even more beneficial than conventional later application.

2.1. Slowing of brain metabolism

When hypothermia was first used in a clinical setting it was presumed that its protective effects were due purely to a slowing of cerebral metabolism, leading to reduced glucose and oxygen consumption. Cerebral metabolism decreases by 6% to 10% for each 1°C reduction in body temperature during cooling.[13,14] This could play a therapeutic effect, but only partially. This mechanism is not the only explanation for the dramatic difference seen despite the positive role of metabolic slowing in neuroprotection.

2.2. Inhibition of apoptosis

Therapeutic hypothermia can also effectively inhibit apoptosis [15-17]Hypothermia inhibits the early stages of the programmed cell death process.[16] Thus, inhibiting apoptosis is another mechanism by which therapeutic hypothermia could influence the ischemia reperfusion injury or secondary injury early on in the disease process.

2.3. Inhibition of excitotoxicity

Excitatory processes play a major role in the pathophysiology of secondary injury post-cardiac arrest.[13] Evidence suggests that hypothermia inhibits these harmful excitatory processes occurring in brain cells during ischemia–reperfusion. Ischemic insult to the brain leads to decrease in Adenosine triphosphate (ATP) supplies.[13] This culminates into an influx of calcium (Ca) into the cell through prolonged glutamate exposure inducing a permanent state of hyperexcitability in the neurons (*excitotoxicity*). All these processes are inhibited by hypothermia very early after injury. Some animal experiments suggest that neuroexcitotoxicity can be blocked or reversed only if the treatment is initiated in the very early stages of the neuroexcitatory cascade.[18-24]

2.4. Antiinflammatory role and decrease in free radical formation

Acute inflammation early after return of spontaneous circulation (ROSC) plays a harmful role in postcardiac arrest, including cytokines, macrophages, neutrophils, and complement activation , leading to free radical formation. Multiple animal experiments and few clinical studies have shown that hypothermia suppresses all these ischemia-induced inflammatory reactions, leading to a significant reduction in free radical formation. [25-28]

2.5. Protection of blood-brain barrier

Ischemia–reperfusion can also lead to significant disruptions in the blood– brain barrier, which can facilitate the subsequent development of brain edema. Mild hypothermia significantly reduces blood– brain barrier disruptions, and also decreases vascular permeability following ischemia–reperfusion, further decreasing edema formation.[29-31]

2.6. Antithrombotic role

The coagulation cascade is also activated with ischemia-reperfusion injury leading to intravascular clot formation resulting in microvascular thrombosis in the brain.[32,33] Therapeutic Hypothermia could be beneficial in this instance since platelets number and function are decreased with temperatures <35°C, and some inhibition of the coagulation cascade develops at temperatures <33°C.[34,35] Vasoconstriction , mediated mainly by thromboxane and endothelin plays a pivotal role in the secondary injury as well. This could also be mitigated by hypothermia [36-38]

3. Clinical evidence

3.1. Out of hospital and ventricular fibrillation cardiac arrest

The first major clinical trials that provided direct evidence of a benefit of therapeutic hypothermia were published in 2002. These studies have indicated that TH with a reduction of body core temperature (T) to 33 °C over 12 to 24 hours has improved survival and neurologic outcome in OHCA patients. The European Hypothermia after Cardiac Arrest Study Group demonstrated an improvement in survival from witnessed V-fib cardiac arrest from 41% to 55% and an improvement in favorable neurologic outcome among survivors from 39% to 55% when TH of 32-34°C was maintained for the first 24 hours post cardiac arrest.39 Bernard demonstrated similar neurologic outcome benefits from 12 hours of TH at 32-34°C induced on the same patient population in Australia.40 Recently, a meta-analysis showed that therapeutic hypothermia is associated with a risk ratio of 1.68 (95% CI,1.29-2.07) favoring a good neurologic outcome when compared with normothermia. The meta-analysis concluded the number needed to treat (NNT) to produce one favorable neurological recovery was 6.41 This would translate to improved neurological recovery in > 10,000 patients per year in the U.S.41 Findings were also reviewed from recent literature on the postresuscitation care of cardiac arrest patients using therapeutic hypothermia as part of nontrial treatment. Although varied in their protocols and outcome reporting, results from published investigations confirmed the findings from the landmark randomized controlled trials, in that the use of therapeutic hypothermia increased survival and favorable neurologic outcome.[42]

3.2. In hospital and non-ventricular fibrillation cardiac arrest

Although ROSC rates are higher in patients with VF and these represent the majority of patients transported to the hospital, many patients still present to the hospital comatose after resuscitation from non-VF arrest. Patients with an initial cardiac rhythm of asystole have a lower rate of survival than patients with VF, because total absence of rhythm is associated with worse underlying causes. Some evidence has now shown that the treatment may be beneficial in cases with non-VF initial rhythm.[43-47] However, other studies involving this patient population did not show outcome benefit. In a recent study of TH after inhospital cardiac arrest (IHCA), 91%of patients had an arrest rhythm of asystole or pulseless electrical activity. No difference in neurological outcome at discharge was detected in these non-shockable IHCA patients treated with TH.[48] Given this increased severity of neurological injury in non-VF arrest patients, the possible role of TH remains uncertain. Given such low rates of recovery after non-VF arrest with the use of TH, a prospective study comparing TH with normothermia in patients with an initial cardiac rhythm asystole or PEA would require very large numbers of patients to get enough power to show improved outcomes, and thus is unlikely that such trials will be conducted.

3.3. Asphyxial causes of cardiac arrest

Suffocation is the second leading cause of death from suicide in the United States, accounting for 22.5% of the 33 300 suicide-related deaths.[49] Victims of near-hanging may carry a poor prognosis even if cardiac arrest has not occurred. Those who suffer cardiac arrest, present with a Glasgow Coma Scale (GCS) of 5 or less, and experience a longer hanging time have the worst prognosis.[50,51]Nearhanging is defined as an unsuccessful attempt at hanging. Victims of near-hanging suffer from strangulation with cerebral ischemia-reperfusion injury rather than a fatal cervical spine injury. Therapeutic Hypothermia has not been prospectively studied in this patient population, and it is doubtful that large randomized, controlled trials comparing TH with normothermia will be conducted. There are few retrospective reviews and case reports and case series on asphyxiated patients with or without cardiac arrests who had good neurologic recovery after therapeutic hypothermia.[52-55] Although it would be difficult to conduct good prospective studies, the compiling case studies, anecdotal evidence, and extrapolated data support the use of therapeutic hypothermia for asphyxial cardiac arrest until more evidence can be obtained.

4. Guidelines

In 2005, guidelines for resuscitation and emergency cardiac care of the European Resuscitation Council and the American Heart Association recommended that the core body temperature of unconscious adult patients with spontaneous circulation after a VF OHCA should be lowered to 32 to 34°C (Class IIA recommendation).[56] Cooling should be started as soon as possible after the arrest and should be continued for at least 12 to 24 hours.

The guidelines note that patients who have had a cardiac arrest due to nonshockable rhythms and patients who have had a cardiac arrest in the hospital may also benefit from induced hypothermia (Class IIB recommendation).[56]

With more evidence and trials showing the feasibility and the evidence supporting TH for cardiac arrest patients, the new guidelines by European Resuscitation Council and the American Heart Association in **2010** recommend that comatose (ie, lack of meaningful response to verbal commands) adult patients with ROSC after out-of-hospital VF cardiac arrest should be cooled to 32°C to 34°C (89.6°F to 93.2°F) for 12 to 24 hours (**Class I**).[57] Induced hypothermia also may be considered for comatose adult patients with ROSC after in-hospital cardiac arrest of any initial rhythm or after out-of-hospital cardiac arrest with an initial rhythm of pulseless electrical activity or asystole (**Class IIb**).[57] Active rewarming should be avoided in comatose patients who spontaneously develop a mild degree of hypothermia (32°C [89.6°F]) after resuscitation from cardiac arrest during the first 48 hours after ROSC. (**Class III**).[57]

5. Cooling methods

5.1. Methods for induction of therapeutic hypothermia

Bernard et al., reported the results of a clinical trial of the rapid infusion of large-volume (30 ml/kg), ice-cold (4°C) lactated ringer's solution in comatose survivors of OHCA. This study found that this approach decreased core temperature by 1.6°C over 25 minutes with no adverse events.[58] Polderman, et al., used in addition to surface cooling, 30ml/kg (mean 2.3 liters) of cold normal saline over 50 minutes that showed similar results.[59] Several small randomized trials, and nonrandomized observational and retrospective trials, looked at pre-hospital cooling initiation for patients with OHCA with large-volume ice-cold (4°C) fluids (discussed in more detail in a separate chapter: **Prehospital Therapeutic Hypothermia for Cardiac Arrest).**[60-68] All these studies documented the safety and feasibility if ice-cold fluids for the rapid induction of therapeutic hypothermia. Other promising methods for induction of hypothermia include transnasal cooling device [69], self-adhesive cooling pads [70], and cranial cooling caps.[71]

5.2. Methods for maintenance of therapeutic hypothermia

An ideal cooling method would be one that will help with rapid induction of cooling, cost-effective, easily implemented, safe, effective, and able to maintain the temperature with minimal variations.

5.2.1. Surface cooling

Ice packs are still used in some centers for induction and maintenance of hypothermia, by applying them to the head, neck, torso and extremities. Disadvantages of this method include slow cooling rate, labor-intensive for the nurses, and wide fluctuations with overshooting and undercooling or unintentional rewarming.[40,72,73]

An effective surface cooling system uses cooling blanket (Arctic Sun, Medivance, Louisville, CO, USA). This technology can cool as fast as 1.2°C per hour through especially designed pads, is radiolucent (can be used during cardiac catheterization), has minimal temperature variation (operates with feedback control), and can perform active controlled rewarming. The pads can be applied easily by the nurses. Disadvantages include expense, possible skin sloughing, and slower cooling rates in very obese people.[72,74]

A promising technology is the Thermosuit System (Life Recovery Systems, Kinnelon, NJ, USA), which surrounds patients directly with cool water and also possesses a feedback control mechanism. Animal studies suggest that it provides a cooling rate of 9.7°C per hour in 30-kg pigs, versus 3.0°C per hour in humans. Disadvantages include expense and hindering appropriate physical exams.[75,76]

5.2.2. Intravascular cooling

The CoolGard System (Alsius, Irvine, CA, USA) is one of the products that uses Intravascular devices. This technology works by exchanging heat through a catheter containing circulating saline at a controlled temperature with a feedback of patient temperature. This technology can cool as fast as 1 to 1.5 °C per hour, is very good at maintaining goal temperature (feedback mechanism) and cal also provide active controlled rewarming. Disadvantages are those of central venous catheters (risks of bleeding, vessel thrombosis, and catheter-related infection). It also requires placement by a physician, which if not readily available, may delay initiation of this important and timely therapy.[77.78]

Although many devices are available to achieve and maintain therapeutic hypothermia, there are no current data recommending one method over another, or comparing them against each other. Several factors need to be taken into consideration, such as patient factors, nursing factors and nurse to patient ratios, and institutional factors when making a decision regarding the optimal method.

6. Conclusion

On the basis of current evidence, comatose (ie, lack of meaningful response to verbal commands) adult patients with ROSC after out-of-hospital VF cardiac arrest should be cooled to 32°C to 34°C (89.6°F to 93.2°F) for 12 to 24 hours, as fast as possible. Therapeutic Hypothermia should be strongly considered for other rhythms, for inhospital arrests, and for cardiac arrest secondary to asphyxia. Intensivists should be familiar with techniques to induce, maintain, and rewarm from therapeutic hypothermia, and select the most appropriate method for a given patient, and institution. Research questions for the future are whether very early cooling, or longer cooling periods (eg, 72 h), or both can further improve outcome.

Author details

Farid Sadaka
Mercy Hospital St Louis/St Louis University ,Critical Care Medicine/Neurocritical Care, St Louis

Acknowledgement

No additional acknowledgements.

Conflicts of interest

The author reports no conflicts of interest.
The author declares that no competing financial interests exist.
The author reports that no potential conflicts of interest exist with any companies/organizations whose products or services may be discussed in this article.

7. References

[1] Stiell IG, Wells GA, Field B, Spaite DW, Nesbitt LP, De Maio VJ, Nichol G, Cousineau D, Blackburn J, Munkley D, Luinstra-Toohey L, Campeau T, Dagnone E, Lyver M; Ontario Prehospital Advanced Life Support Study Group (2004) Advanced cardiac life support in out-of-hospital cardiac arrest. N Engl J Med 351:647- 656.

[2] Keenan SP, Dodek P, Martin C, Priestap F, Norena M, Wong H (2007) Variation in length of intensive care unit stay after cardiac arrest: where you are is as important as who you are. Crit Care Med 35: 836–841.

[3] Mashiko K, Otsuka T, Shimazaki S, Kohama A, Kamishima G, Katsurada K, Sawada Y, Matsubara I, Yamaguchi K (2002) An outcome study of out-of-hospital cardiac arrest using the Utstein template: a Japanese experience. Resuscitation 55:241–246.

[4] Nolan JP, Laver SR, Welch CA, Harrison DA, Gupta V, Rowan K (2007) Outcome following admission to UK intensive care units after cardiac arrest: a secondary analysis of the ICNARC Case Mix Programme Database. Anaesthesia 62:1207–1216.

[5] Langhelle A, Tyvold SS, Lexow K, Hapnes SA, Sunde K, Steen PA (2003) In-hospital factors associated with improved outcome after out-ofhospital cardiac arrest: a comparison between four regions in Norway. Resuscitation 56:247–263.

[6] Herlitz J, Engdahl J, Svensson L, Angquist KA, Silfverstolpe J, Holmberg S (2006) Major differences in 1-month survival between hospitals in Sweden among initial survivors of out-of-hospital cardiac arrest. Resuscitation 70:404–409.

[7] Neumar RW, Nolan JP, Adrie C, Aibiki M, Berg RA, Böttiger BW, Callaway C, Clark RSB, Geocadin RG, Jauch EC, Kern KB, Laurent I, Longstreth WT Jr, Merchant RM, Morley P, Morrison LJ, Nadkarni V, Peberdy MA, Rivers EP, Rodriguez-Nunez A, Sellke FW, Spaulding C, Sunde K, Vanden Hoek T (2008) Post– cardiac arrest syndrome: epidemiology, pathophysiology, treatment, and prognostication: a consensus statement from the International Liaison Committee on Resuscitation (American Heart Association, Australian and New Zealand Council on Resuscitation, European Resuscitation Council, Heart and Stroke Foundation of Canada, InterAmerican Heart Foundation, Resuscitation Council of Asia, and the Resuscitation Council of Southern Africa); the American Heart Association Emergency Cardiovascular Care Committee; the Council on Cardiovascular Surgery and Anesthesia; the Council on Cardiopulmonary, Perioperative, and Critical Care; the Council on Clinical Cardiology; and the Stroke Council. Circulation 118:2452–2483.

[8] Eisenberg MS, Mengert TJ (2001) Cardiac Resuscitation. N Engl J Med 334: 1304-1313.

[9] Bunch TJ, White RD, Smith GE, Hodge DO, Gersh BJ, Hammill SC, Shen WK, Packer DL (1998) Long-term subjective memory function in ventricular fibrillation out-of-hospital cardiac arrest survivors resuscitated by early defibrillation. Resuscitation 36:111-122.

[10] Laver S, Farrow C, Turner D, Nolan J (2004) Mode of death after admission to an intensive care unit following cardiac arrest. Intensive Care Med 30:2126 –2128.

[11] Jacobs I, Nadkarni V, Bahr J, Berg RA, Billi JE, Bossaert L, Cassan P, Coovadia A, D'Este K, Finn J, Halperin H, Handley A, Herlitz J, Hickey R, Idris A, Kloeck W, Larkin GL,

Mancini ME, Mason P, Mears G, Monsieurs K, Montgomery W, Morley P, Nichol G, Nolan J, Okada K, Perlman J, Shuster M, Steen PA, Sterz F, Tibballs J, Timerman S, Truitt T, Zideman D; International Liaison Committee on Resuscitation (2004) Cardiac arrest and cardiopulmonary resuscitation outcome reports: update and simplification of the Utstein templates for resuscitation registries: a statement for healthcare professionals from a task force of the International Liaison Committee on Resuscitation (American Heart Association, European Resuscitation Council, Australian Resuscitation Council, New Zealand Resuscitation Council, Heart and Stroke Foundation of Canada, InterAmerican Heart Foundation, Resuscitation Council of Southern Africa). Resuscitation 63:233–249.

[12] Polderman KH (2008) Induced hypothermia and fever control for prevention and treatment of neurological injuries. Lancet 371: 1955–1969.

[13] Small DL, Morley P, Buchan AM (1999) Biology of ischemic cerebral cell death. Prog Cardiovasc Dis 42:185–207.

[14] Hagerdal M, Harp J, Nilsson L, Siesjö BK (1975) The effect of induced hypothermia upon oxygen consumption in the rat brain. J Neurochem 24:311–316.

[15] Povlishock JT, Buki A, Koiziumi H, Stone J, Okonkwo DO (1999) Initiating mechanisms involved in the pathobiology of traumatically induced axonal injury and interventions targeted at blunting their progression. Acta Neurochir Suppl (Wien) 73:15–20

[16] Xu L, Yenari MA, Steinberg GK, Giffard RG (2002) Mild hypothermia reduces apoptosis of mouse neurons in vitro early in the cascade. J Cereb Blood Flow Metab 22:21–28

[17] Ning XH, Chen SH, Xu CS, Li L, Yao LY, Qian K, Krueger JJ, Hyyti OM, Portman MA (2002) Hypothermic protection of the ischemic heart via alterations in apoptotic pathways as assessed by gene array analysis. J Appl Physiol 92:2200–2207

[18] Siesjo BK, Bengtsson F, Grampp W, Theander S (1989) Calcium, excitotoxins, and neuronal death in brain. Ann NY Acad Sci 568: 234–251.

[19] Leker RR, Shohami E (2002) Cerebral ischemia and trauma—different etiologies yet similar mechanisms: Neuroprotective opportunities. Brain Res Brain Res Rev 39: 55–73

[20] Dempsey RJ, Combs DJ, Maley ME, Cowen DE, Roy MW, Donaldson DL (1987) Moderate hypothermia reduces postischemic edema development and leukotriene production. Neurosurgery 21:177–181.

[21] Globus MY-T, Alonso O, Dietrich WD, Busto R, Ginsberg MD (1995) Glutamate release and free radical production following brain injury: Effects of posttraumatic hypothermia. J Neurochem 65:1704–1711.

[22] Busto R, Globus MY, Dietrich WD, Martinez E, Valdés I, Ginsberg MD (1989) Effect of mild hypothermia on ischemia-induced release of neurotransmitters and free fatty acids in rat brain. Stroke 20:904–910.

[23] Takata K, Takeda Y, Morita K (2005) Effects of hypothermia for a short period on histological outcome and extracellular glutamate concentration during and after cardiac arrest in rats. Crit Care Med 33: 1340–1345.

[24] Kuboyama K, Safar P, Radovsky A, Tisherman SA, Stezoski SW, Alexander H (1993) Delay in cooling negates the beneficial effect of mild resuscitative cerebral hypothermia

after cardiac arrest in dogs: A prospective, randomized study. Crit Care Med 21:1348–1358.

[25] Aibiki M, Maekawa S, Ogura S, Kinoshita Y, Kawai N, Yokono S (1999) Effect of moderate hypothermia on systemic and internal jugular plasma IL-6 levels after traumatic brain injury in humans. J Neurotrauma 16:225–232.

[26] Schmidt OI, Heyde CE, Ertel W, Stahel PF (2005) Closed head injury—an inflammatory disease? Brain Res Brain Res Rev 48: 388–399.

[27] Kimura A, Sakurada S, Ohkuni H, Todome Y, Kurata K (2002) Moderate hypothermia delays proinflammatory cytokine production of human peripheral blood mononuclear cells. Crit Care Med 30:1499–1502.

[28] Dietrich WD, Chatzipanteli K, Vitarbo E, Wada K, Kinoshita K (2004) The role of inflammatory processes in the pathophysiology and treatment of brain and spinal cord trauma. Acta Neurochir Suppl 89:69–74.

[29] Chi OZ, Liu X, Weiss HR (2001) Effects of mild hypothermia on blood- brain barrier disruption during isoflurane or pentobarbital anesthesia. Anesthesiology 95:933–938.

[30] Smith SL, Hall ED (1996) Mild pre- and posttraumatic hypothermia attenuates blood–brain barrier damage following controlled cortical impact injury in the rat. J Neurotrauma 13:1–9.

[31] Jurkovich GJ, Pitt RM, Curreri PW, Granger DN (1988) Hypothermia prevents increased capillary permeability following ischemia–reperfusion injury. J Surg Res 44:514–521.

[32] Bo¨ttiger BW, Motsch J, Bohrer H, Böker T, Aulmann M, Nawroth PP, Martin E (1995) Activation of blood coagulation after cardiac arrest is not balanced adequately by activation of endogenous fibrinolysis. Circulation 92:2572–2578.

[33] Gando S, Kameue T, Nanzaki S, Nakanishi Y (1997) Massive fibrin formation with consecutive impairment of fibrinolysis in patients with out-of-hospital cardiac arrest. Thromb Haemost 77:278–282.

[34] Michelson AD, MacGregor H, Barnard MR, Kestin AS, Rohrer MJ, Valeri CR (1994) Hypothermia-induced reversible platelet dysfunction. Thromb Haemost 71:633–640.

[35] Valeri CR, MacGregor H, Cassidy G, Tinney R, Pompei F (1995) Effects of temperature on bleeding time and clotting time in normal male and female volunteers. Crit Care Med 23: 698–704.

[36] Chen ST, Hsu CY, Hogan EL, Halushka PV, Linet OI, Yatsu FM (1986) Thromboxane, prostacyclin, and leukotrienes in cerebral ischemia. Neurology 36: 466–470.

[37] Maekawa S, Aibiki M, Ogura S (1997) Mild hypothermia suppresses thromboxane B2 production in brain-injured patients. In: The Immune Consequences of Trauma, Shock and Sepsis. Mechanisms and Therapeutic Approaches. Faist E (Ed). Bologna, Italy, Monduzzi Editore pp 135–138.

[38] Aibiki M, Maekawa S, Yokono S (2000) Moderate hypothermia improves imbalances of thromboxane A2 and prostaglandin I2 production after traumatic brain injury in humans. Crit Care Med 28:3902–3906.

[39] Hypothermia After Cardiac Arrest Study Group (2002) Mild therapeutic hypothermia to improve the neurologic outcome after cardiac arrest. N Engl J Med 346:549 –556.

[40] Bernard SA, Gray TW, Buist MD, Jones BM, Silvester W, Gutteridge G, Smith K (2002) Treatment of comatose survivors of out-of-hospital cardiac arrest with induced hypothermia. N Engl J Med 346:557–563.

[41] Holzer M, Bernard SA, Hachimi-Idrissi S, Roine RO, Sterz F, Müllner M; Collaborative Group on Induced Hypothermia for Neuroprotection After Cardiac Arrest (2005) Hypothermia for neuroprotection after cardiac arrest: systematic review and individual patient data meta-analysis. Crit Care Med 33:414–418.

[42] Sagalyn E, Band RA, Gaieski DF Abella BS (2009) Therapeutic hypothermia after cardiac arrest in clinical practice: review and compilation of recent experiences. Crit Care Med 37(7 Suppl):S223-6.

[43] Oddo M, Schaller MD, Feihl F, Ribordy V, Liaudet L (2006) From evidence to clinical practice: effective implementation of therapeutic hypothermia to improve patient outcome after cardiac arrest. Crit Care Med 34: 1865–1873.

[44] Sunde K, Pytte M, Jacobsen D, Mangschau A, Jensen LP, Smedsrud C, Draegni T, Steen PA (2007) Implementation of a standardised treatment protocol for post resuscitation care after out-of-hospital cardiac arrest. Resuscitation 73:29 –39.

[45] Busch M, Soreide E, Lossius HM, Lexow K, Dickstein K (2006) Rapid implementation of therapeutic hypothermia in comatose out-of-hospital cardiac arrest survivors. Acta Anaesthesiol Scand 50:1277–1283.

[46] Arrich J; European Resuscitation Council Hypothermia After Cardiac Arrest Registry Study Group (2007) Clinical application of mild therapeutic hypothermia after cardiac arrest. Crit Care Med 35:1041–1047.

[47] Holzer M, Müllner M, Sterz F, Robak O, Kliegel A, Losert H, Sodeck G, Uray T, Zeiner A, Laggner AN (2006) Efficacy and safety of endovascular cooling after cardiac arrest: cohort study and Bayesian approach. Stroke 37:1792–1797.

[48] Kory P, Fukunaga M, Mathew JP, Singh B, Szainwald L, Mosak J, Marks M, Berg D, Saadia M, Katz A, Mayo PH (2012) Outcomes of Mild Therapeutic Hypothermia After In-Hospital Cardiac Arrest. Neurocrit Care [Epub ahead of print].

[49] Statistical abstract of the U.S. In: Bureau USC, ed 2005-2006.

[50] Matsuyama T, Okuchi K, Tadahiko S, Murao Y (2004) Prognostic factors in hanging injuries. Am J Emerg Med 22(3):207-10.

[51] Penney DJ, Stewart P (2002) Prognostic outcome indicators following hanging injuries. Resuscitation 54:27-9.

[52] Borgquist O, Friberg H (2009) Therapeutic hypothermia for comatose survivors after near-hanging—a retrospective analysis. Resuscitation 80:210-2.

[53] Jehle D, Meyer M, Gemme S (2010) Beneficial response to mild therapeutic hypothermia for comatose survivors of near-hanging. Am J Emerg Med 28:390.e1-e3.

[54] Howell MA, Guly HR (1996) Near hanging presenting to an accident and emergency department. Am J Accid Emerg Med 13:135-6.

[55] Sadaka F, Wood MP, Cox M (2012) Therapeutic hypothermia for a comatose survivor of near-hanging. Am J Emerg Med 30(1):251.e1-2.

[56] 2005 American Heart Association Guidelines for Cardiopulmonary Resuscitation and Emergency Cardiovascular Care Part 7.5: Postresuscitation Support. Circulation 112:IV-84–IV- 88.

[57] Peberdy MA, Callaway CW, Neumar RW, Geocadin RG, Zimmerman JL, Donnino M, Gabrielli A, Silvers SM, Zaritsky AL, Merchant R, Vanden Hoek TL, Kronick SL (2010) Part 9: post– cardiac arrest care: 2010 American Heart Association Guidelines for Cardiopulmonary Resuscitation and Emergency Cardiovascular Care. Circulation 122(suppl 3):S768 –S786.

[58] Bernard S, Buist M, Monteiro O, Smith K (2003) Induced hypothermia using large volume, ice-cold intravenous fluid in comatose survivors of out-of- hospital cardiac arrest: a preliminary report. Resuscitation 56:9 –13.

[59] Polderman KH, Rijnsburger ER, Peerdeman SM, Girbes AR (2005) Induction of hypothermia in patients with various types of neurologic injury with use of large volumes of ice-cold intravenous fluid. Crit Care Med 33:2744 –2751.

[60] Kim F, Olsufka M, Longstreth WT Jr, Maynard C, Carlbom D, Deem S, Kudenchuk P, Copass MK, Cobb LA (2007) Pilot randomized clinical trial of prehospital induction of mild hypothermia in out ofhospital cardiac arrest patients with a rapid infusion of 4 degrees C normal saline. Circulation 115:3064-70.

[61] Kämäräinen A, Virkkunen I, Tenhunen J, Yli-Hankala A, Silfvast T (2009) Prehospital therapeutic hypothermia for comatose survivors of cardiac arrest: a randomized controlled trial. Acta Anaesthesiol Scand 53:900-7.

[62] Bernard SA, Smith K, Cameron P, Masci K, Taylor DM, Cooper DJ, Kelly AM, Silvester W; Rapid Infusion of Cold Hartmanns (RICH) Investigators (2010) Induction of therapeutic hypothermia by paramedics after resuscitation from out-of-hospital ventricular fibrillation cardiac arrest: a randomized controlled trial. Circulation 122(7):737-42.

[63] Bernard SA, Smith K, Cameron P, Masci K, Taylor DM, Cooper DJ, Kelly AM, Silvester W; Rapid Infusion of Cold Hartmanns (RICH) Investigators (2012) Induction of prehospital therapeutic hypothermia after resuscitation from nonventricular fibrillation cardiac arrest. Crit Care Med 40(3):747-53.

[64] Virkkunen I, Yli-Hankala A, Silfvast T (2004) Induction of therapeutic hypothermia after cardiac arrest in prehospital patients using ice-cold Ringer's solution: a pilot study. Resuscitation. 62:299-302.

[65] Hammer L, Vitrat F, Savary D, Debaty G, Santre C, Durand M, Dessertaine G, Timsit JF (2009) Immediate prehospital hypothermia protocol in comatose survivors of out-of-hospital cardiac arrest. Am J Emerg Med. 27:570-3.

[66] Kämäräinen A, Virkkunen I, Tenhunen J, Yli-Hankala A, Silfvast T (2008) Induction of therapeutic hypothermia during prehospital CPR using ice-cold intravenous fluid. Resuscitation 79:205-11.

[67] Bruel C, Parienti JJ, Marie W, Arrot X, Daubin C, Du Cheyron D, Massetti M, Charbonneau P (2008) Mild hypothermia during advanced life support: a preliminary study in out-of-hospital cardiac arrest. Crit Care 12:R31.

[68] Garrett JS, Studnek JR, Blackwell T, Vandeventer S, Pearson DA, Heffner AC, Reades R (2011) The association between intra-arrest therapeutic hypothermia and return of spontaneous circulation among individuals experiencing out of hospital cardiac arrest. Resuscitation 82(1):21-5.

[69] Castre´n M, Nordberg P, Svensson L, Taccone F, Vincent JL, Desruelles D, Eichwede F, Mols P, Schwab T, Vergnion M, Storm C, Pesenti A, Pachl J, Gue´risse F, Elste T, Roessler M, Fritz H, Durnez P, Busch H-J, Inderbitzen B, Barbut D (2010) Intra-arrest transnasal evaporative cooling: a randomized, prehospital, multicenter study (PRINCE: Pre-ROSC Intra-Nasal Cooling Effectiveness). Circulation 122:729–736.

[70] Uray T, Malzer R, on behalf of the Vienna Hypothermia After Cardiac Arrest (HACA) Study Group (2008) Out-of-hospital surface cooling to induce mild hypothermia in human cardiac arrest: A feasibility trial. Resuscitation 77:331-338.

[71] Storm C, Schefold JC, Kerner T, Schmidbauer W, Gloza J, Krueger A, Jörres A, Hasper D (2008) Prehospital cooling with hypothermia caps (PreCoCa): a feasibility study. Clin Res Cardiol 97:768-72.

[72] Janata A, Holzer M (2009) Hypothermia after cardiac arrest. Prog Cardiovasc Dis 52(2):168 –79.

[73] Merchant RM, Abella BS, Peberdy MA, Soar J, Ong ME, Schmidt GA, Becker LB, Vanden Hoek TL (2006) Therapeutic hypothermia after cardiac arrest: unintentional overcooling is common using ice packs and conventional cooling blankets. Crit Care Med 34:S490–S494.

[74] Haugk M, Sterz F, Grassberger M, Uray T, Kliegel A, Janata A, Richling N, Herkner H, Laggner AN (2007) Feasibility and efficacy of a new non-invasive surface cooling device in post-resuscitation intensive care medicine. Resuscitation 75(1):76–81.

[75] Schratter A, Weihs W, Holzer M, Janata A, Behringer W, Losert UM, Ohley WJ, Schock RB, Sterz F (2007) External cardiac defibrillation during wet surface cooling in pigs. Am J Emerg Med 25(4):420–4.

[76] Howes D, Ohley W, Dorian P, Klock C, Freedman R, Schock R, Krizanac D, Holzer M (2010) Rapid induction of therapeutic hypothermia using convective-immersion surface cooling: safety, efficacy and outcomes. Resuscitation 81(4):388 –92.

[77] Holzer M, Mullner M, Sterz F, Robak O, Kliegel A, Losert H, Sodeck G, Uray T, Zeiner A, Laggner AN (2006) Efficacy and safety of endovascular cooling after cardiac arrest: cohort study and Bayesian approach. Stroke 37(7):1792–7.

[78] Al-Senani FM, Graffagnino C, Grotta JC, Saiki R, Wood D, Chung W, Palmer G, Collins KA (2004) A prospective, multicenter pilot study to evaluate the feasibility and safety of using the CoolGard System and Icy catheter following cardiac arrest. Resuscitation 62(2):143–50.

Chapter 3

Prehospital Therapeutic Hypothermia for Cardiac Arrest

Farid Sadaka

Additional information is available at the end of the chapter

http://dx.doi.org/10.5772/49049

1. Introduction

In the era before Therapeutic Hypothermia (TH) was recommended and used as a therapeutic modality for out-of-hospital cardiac arrest (OHCA) patients, reported data suggests in-hospital mortality exceeded 58%.[1,2,3,4,5,6] Mortality after a sudden and unexpected cardiac arrest (CA) is high, and the chance of survival to hospital discharge has, until recently, remained unchanged.[7] In one report, OHCA in the U.S. has a mortality rate greater than 90% which results in more than 300,000 deaths per year.[8] Those who survive the devastating event, often retain a hypoxic brain injury and a permanently incapacitating neurologic deficit.[9] Studies of patients who survived to ICU admission but subsequently died in the hospital, brain injury was the cause of death in 68% after out-of-hospital cardiac arrest and in 23% after in-hospital cardiac arrest.[10,11]

Recent studies have indicated that TH with a reduction of body core temperature (T) to 33 °C over 12 to 24 hours has improved survival and neurologic outcome in OHCA patients. In 2002, the European Hypothermia after Cardiac Arrest Study Group demonstrated an improvement in survival from witnessed V-fib cardiac arrest from 41% to 55% and an improvement in favorable neurologic outcome among survivors from 39% to 55% when TH of 32-34°C was maintained for the first 24 hours post cardiac arrest.[12] Bernard demonstrated similar neurologic outcome benefits from 12 hours of TH at 32-34°C induced on the same patient population in Australia.[13] Recently, a meta-analysis showed that therapeutic hypothermia is associated with a risk ratio of 1.68 (95% CI,1.29-2.07) favoring a good neurologic outcome when compared with normothermia. The meta-analysis concluded the number needed to treat (NNT) to produce one favorable neurological recovery was 6.[14] This would translate to improved neurological recovery in > 10,000 patients per year in the U.S.[14] Also, recent evidence has now shown that the treatment is beneficial in cases with non-VF initial rhythm.[15,16,17,18,19].

Current resuscitation guidelines of the International Liaison Committee on Resuscitation (ILCOR) recommend induction of TH in post-cardiac arrest patients.[7] In 2005 and then upgraded in 2010, the American Heart Association Advanced Cardiac Life Support Guidelines recommended that "unconscious adult patients with ROSC after out-of-hospital cardiac arrest should be cooled to 32 to 34°C for 12-24 hours…."[20,21]. The guidelines identified the need for cooling to occur in the pre-hospital arena, noting that hypothermia "should probably be initiated as soon as possible after ROSC…."

2. Basic science

A cascade of destructive events and processes begins at the cellular level in the minutes to hours following an initial injury. These processes, the result of ischemia and reperfusion, may continue for hours to many days after the initial injury.[22]

When hypothermia was first used in a clinical setting it was presumed that its protective effects were due purely to a slowing of cerebral metabolism, leading to reduced glucose and oxygen consumption. Cerebral metabolism decreases by 6% to 10% for each 1°C reduction in body temperature during cooling.[23,24] This could play a therapeutic effect, but only partially. Therapeutic hypothermia can also effectively inhibit apoptosis. [25-27]Hypothermia inhibits the early stages of the programmed cell death process.[26] Thus, inhibiting apoptosis is another mechanism by which therapeutic hypothermia could influence the ischemia reperfusion injury or secondary injury early on in the disease process. Excitatory processes play a major role in the pathophysiology of secondary injury post-cardiac arrest.[23] Evidence suggests that hypothermia inhibits these harmful excitatory processes occurring in brain cells during ischemia–reperfusion. Ischemic insult to the brain leads to decrease in Adenosine triphosphate (ATP) supplies.[23] This culminates into an influx of calcium (Ca) into the cell through prolonged glutamate exposure inducing a permanent state of hyperexcitability in the neurons (*excitotoxicity*). All these processes are inhibited by hypothermia very early after injury. Some animal experiments suggest that neuroexcitotoxicity can be blocked or reversed only if the treatment is initiated in the very early stages of the neuroexcitatory cascade.[28-34] Acute inflammation early after ROSC plays a harmful role in postcardiac arrest, including cytokines, macrophages, neutrophils, and complement activation, leading to free radical formation. Multiple animal experiments and few clinical studies have shown that hypothermia suppresses all these ischemia-induced inflammatory reactions, leading to a significant reduction in free radical formation. [35-38] Ischemia–reperfusion can also lead to significant disruptions in the blood– brain barrier, which can facilitate the subsequent development of brain edema. Mild hypothermia significantly reduces blood– brain barrier disruptions, and also decreases vascular permeability following ischemia–reperfusion, further decreasing edema formation.[39-41] The coagulation cascade is also activated with ischemia-reperfusion injury leading to intravascular clot formation resulting in microvascular thrombosis in the brain. [42,43] Therapeutic Hypothermia could be beneficial in this instance since platelets number and function are decreased with temperatures <35°C, and some inhibition of the coagulation cascade develops at temperatures <33°C.[44,45] Vasoconstriction, mediated mainly by thromboxane and endothelin plays a pivotal role in the secondary injury as well. This could also be mitigated by hypothermia [46-48]

It is crucial to note that all of these processes after ischemic-reperfusion injury in the brain are temperature dependent; they are all stimulated by fever, and can all be mitigated or blocked by hypothermia. Since most of these processes start within minutes to hours after the injury, then application of hypothermia earlier might be even more beneficial than conventional later application. This has been the premise behind prehospital cooling.

3. Animal studies

Animal studies demonstrate a benefit of very early cooling either during CPR or within 15 minutes of ROSC when cooling is maintained for only a short duration (1 to 2 hours). Equivalent neuroprotection was produced in a rat model of cardiac arrest when a 24-hour period of cooling was either initiated at the time of ROSC or delayed by 1 hour. In a gerbil forebrain ischemia model, sustained neuroprotection was achieved when hypothermia was initiated at 1, 6, or 12 hours after reperfusion and maintained for 48 hours; however, neuroprotection did decrease when the start of therapy was delayed. Mice receiving intra-arrest cooling had more favorable hemodynamic and neurological outcomes compared with normothermic controls with earlier reperfusion time. In another model, Dogs that received hypothermia treatment within 10 minutes of onset of VF had significantly better neurological outcomes than those that received it after 20 minutes of VF. [49-53]

4. Human studies

Bernard et al., reported the results of a clinical trial of the rapid infusion of large-volume (30 ml/kg), ice-cold (4°C) lactated ringer's solution in comatose survivors of OHCA. This study found that this approach decreased core temperature by 1.6°C over 25 minutes with no adverse events.[54] Polderman, et al., used in addition to surface cooling, 30ml/kg (mean 2.3 liters) of cold normal saline over 50 minutes that showed similar results.[55] Several small randomized trials[56-59], and nonrandomized observational and retrospective trials [60-66], looked at pre-hospital cooling initiation for patients with OHCA.

The first randomized controlled trial (RCT) of pre-hospital cooling using large volume ice chilled fluid (LVICF) was reported by Kim et al. in 2007. Adult victims of non-traumatic cardiac arrest regardless of the initial rhythm were randomized either to field cooling or conventional treatment. In EMS before hospital arrival, patients assigned to the treatment group were infused up to 2L of 4°C normal saline as soon as possible after resuscitation from out-of-hospital cardiac arrest. A total of 125 patients were randomized to receive standard care with or without intravenous cooling. Among survivors to hospital admission, a significant esophageal temperature decrease of 1.24°C was observed in the treatment group compared to a 0.10°C increase in the control group. The authors report no increase in the number of adverse events associated with field cooling.[56] Kämäräinen et al conducted a similar safety trial in 2009; patients were cooled using LVICF and compared to patients

Trial	Cooling method	Randomized-controlled	Number of patients	Temperature measurement site	Complications
Kim et al 2007	LVICF	YES	125	esophageal	No difference
Kämäräinen et al 2009	LVICF	YES	37	nasopharyngeal	No difference
Bernard et al 2010	LVICF	YES	234	Tympanic	No difference
Bernard et al 2011	LVICF	YES	163	Tympanic	No difference
Castren et al 2010	Transnasal cooling	YES	200	Tympanic and core	No difference
Callaway et al 2002	Ice Packs	NO	22	Nasopharyngeal esophageal	No
Virkkunen et al 2004	LVICF	NO	13	Esophageal	1 hypotension
Uray et al 2008	Cooling pads	NO	15	Esophageal	No
Hammer et al 2009	LVICF	NO	99	Rectal	No difference
Storm et al 2008	Cooling cap	NO	45	Tympanic	No
Kämäräinen et al 2008	LVICF	NO	17	Nasopharyngeal	5 Re- arrests
Bruel et al 2008	LVICF	NO	33	Esophageal	1 Pulmonary edema
Garrett et al 2011	ICF (2000ml)	NO	551	Core	No difference

LVICF; large volume ice chilled fluid, ICF; ice chilled fluid

Table 1. Clinical Trials on prehospital cooling

received conventional fluid therapy. Of 44 patients screened, 19 were cooled using LVICF and 18 patients received conventional fluid therapy. LVICF resulted in a mean decrease in nasopharyngeal temperature of 1.5 °C. At the time of hospital admission, the mean nasopharyngeal temperature was markedly lower in the hypothermia group compared to the control group; 34.1°C vs. 35.2°C, respectively. Otherwise, there were no significant differences between the groups regarding safety parameters.[57] Bernard et al, in 2010, randomized 234 patients with an initial rhythm of Ventricular fibrillation (VF) to treatment group to receive 2L of LVICF by paramedics or to the control group to be cooled after hospital admission.[58] Patients allocated to paramedic cooling received a median of 1900 mL of ice-cold fluid. This resulted in a mean decrease in core temperature of 0.8°C. However, patients in both prehospital TH and control groups had equivalent temperatures at 60 minutes after hospital arrival (34.7°C). They did not demonstrate any improvement in survival to hospital discharge among prehospital-cooled patients when compared with patients receiving TH initiated in the hospital. In a subsequent study, Bernard et al randomized 163 patients with an initial rhythm of non-VF to either pre-hospital cooling using a rapid infusion of LVICF or cooling after hospital admission.[59] Patients allocated to prehospital cooling received a median of 1500 ml of ice-cold fluid. This resulted in a mean decrease in core temperature of 1.4°C compared with 0.2°C in hospital cooled patients. Although the planned duration of TH in both groups was 24 hours, both groups received a mean of 15 hours cooling in the hospital and only 7 patients in each group were cooled for 24 hours. There was no difference in outcomes at hospital discharge with favorable outcome in the pre-hospital cooled patients, compared with in the hospital cooled patients. In another randomized, controlled trial in 2010, Castren et al examined the use of transnasal cooling in the prehospital setting after ROSC, using an experimental portable delivery device.[60] They showed that transnasal cooling was safe and effective during arrest, with a rapid onset of TH in the prehospital setting. Although they did not demonstrate a statistically significant difference in survival to hospital discharge, there was a trend to increased survival in the transnasal cooling group compared with the control group (43.8% vs. 31.0%; $p = 0.26$). In a subset of patients who had CPR initiated within 10 minutes of collapse, there was a statistically significant difference in those who survived in the cooled group versus the control group (56.5% vs. 29.4%; $p = 0.04$) and those who were neurologically intact (43.5% vs. 17.6%; $p = 0.03$).

Callaway et al in 2002 applied ice to the heads and necks of 9 patients during CPR, and compared this to a control group of 13 patients.[61] There was no difference in the rate of cooling in this study. Virkkunen et al, in 2004 reported a feasibility study using post ROSC infusion of 30 ml/kg LVICF after ROSC. In this cohort of thirteen patients, a significant decrease in esophageal temperature was observed, with a mean decrease of 1.9°C compared to the temperature prior to the onset of infusion.[62] A transient episode of hypotension was observed in one patient, but otherwise the treatment was well tolerated. In 2008, Uray et al used self-adhesive cooling pads to induce cooling in the prehospital setting after ROSC in 15 patients.[63] The rate of cooling was 3.3 °C/h; the target temperature (33 to 34°C) was reached in hospital after approximately 91 minutesfrom the time of ROSC. This study also showed that prehospital cooling was feasible and no adverse events were observed. In a retrospective review of 22 patients cooled using LVICF in the prehospital setting following ROSC compared to 77 conventionally treated patients in 2009, Hammer et al showed prehospital cooling to be easible and safe with a mean cooling rate of -1.7 C/h and no significant increase in the rate of adverse effects in the cooling group compared to the conventional group. [64] Storm et al, in 2008, studied the feasibility of a cranial cooling cap in the prehospital setting initiated after ROSC in 20 patients compared to 25 patients serving as a non-randomized control group.[65] A 1.1°C decrease in tympanic temperature was observed in the treatment group. Also, in 2008, Kämäräinen et al enrolled 17 patients in a nonrandomized study where paramedics initiated cooling using LVICF during CPR and after ROSC with a target temperature of 33°C.[66] The mean infused volume was 1571 ± 517 ml and resulted in a mean admission temperature of 33.83 ± 0.77°C (1.34°C decrease compared to initial nasopharyngeal temperature). There were no major adverse events. In a similar study, Bruel et al enrolled 33 patients out of whom 20 patients had ROSC.[67] A mean esophageal temperature decrease of 2.1°C was observed. Pulmonary edema occurred in one patient. No other major adverse events occurred. In 2011, Garrett et al performed a retrospective analysis of individuals experiencing OHCA whereby six months into the study a prehospital intraarrest TH (IATH) protocol was instituted.[68] In this protocol, patients received 2000 ml of ICF directly after obtaining intravenous access. 551 patients were analysed. Rates of prehospital ROSC were 36.5% versus 26.9% (OR 1.83; 95% CI 1.19–2.81) in patients who received IATH versus normothermic resuscitation respectively. While the frequency of survival to hospital admission and discharge were increased among those receiving IATH, the differences did not reach statistical significance.The secondary analysis found a linear association between the amount of cold saline infused and the likelihood of prehospital ROSC. They concluded that the infusion of 2000 ml of ICF during the intra-arrest period may improve rate of ROSC.

These studies are either underpowered or due to study design do not allow conclusions regarding effects on outcome to be drawn, but the safety and feasibility of early cooling was demonstrated. Another major limitation in most of these studies is that TH is not systematically continued in the post resuscitation care occurring in-hospital. Therefore, it is not possible to evaluate the benefits of pre-hospital cooling alone, as the effect of TH has been shown to necessitate a cooling period of at least 12 to 24 hours.

5. Methods for induction of prehospital therapeutic hypothermia

Most of the trials described above (Table 1) used LVICF for induction of TH in the prehospital setting. All the studies that used LVICF showed that this method for cooling is safe and feasible. However, LVICF may portend some potential problems. In one study on cold fluids, it was shown that chilled fluids begin to warm during transit through intravenous tubing, but the rate was not rapid enough to be deemed potentially clinically significant.[69] In addition, in some instances, time to transport from the field to the emergency department may be too short for LVICF to have a significant cooling effect. In a study by Spaite et al on prehospital cardiac arrest, the time to transport from the field to the hospital was about 7 minutes.[70] In the study by Bernard et al above, 52% of the patients did not receive the goal of 2 L chilled saline because the transport time to the hospital was < 20 minutes.[58] EMS systems with short transport times may not benefit from prehospital TH methods, esp chilled fluids, as much as systems that need longer time to get to their respective facilities. Another cooling method, used by Castren et al was transnasal cooling, with a machine that employs evaporation of an inert liquid sprayed in the posterior nasopharynx.[60] They did show that this method of transnasal cooling was safe and effective during arrest, with a rapid onset of TH in the prehospital setting. However, it is expensive and not widely available at this point. Another method used was cooling pads by Uray et al.[63] They used prechilled cooling pads that were stored in an insulated box with a cooling battery. They were able to achieve target temperature within about 50 minutes with only mild dermal erythema, which resolved soon after removal of the pads. Storm et al used cooling caps that proved feasible and with no significant adverse events.[65] Other promising new technologies include chilled perfluorocarbons and saline/ice "slurries", that are still at level of animal experimentation.[71,72]

6. Complications and problems with prehospital therapeutic hypothermia

The usual side effects pertaining to therapeutic hypothermia in general like arrhythmias, electrolyte abnormalities, bleeding, infection and other complications could also happen here, however these are discussed in a previous chapter. In this section, I will discuss the complications and problems pertinent to the prehospital phase of hypothermia induction. Overcooling is a potential problem in the field. It is very important to avoid overcooling below the target range because adverse events likely increase when patients are cooled to < 32°C.[73,74] In a retrospective review, investigators showed that unintentional overcooling below target temperature is common, and concluded that improved mechanisms for temperature control are required to prevent potentially deleterious complications of more profound hypothermia.[75] I also add that effective and accurate methods for prehospital temperature monitoring is important, such as tympanic or esophageal temperature monitors. Another important complication is shivering, especially in the EMS with some limitations on use of antishivering medications, such as neuromascular blockers and some sedatives. One important potential problem is the interference of inducing TH in the field with the actual CPR and ACLS ongoing on the patient. Some providers believe that basic resuscitation care should be prioritized over induction of TH, especially with no proven outcome benefit of prehospital TH. A survey of EMS physicians on the implementation rate of prehospital cooling in the United States reported that the most common barriers to prehospital hypothermia are the lack of ideal equipment and space in EMS vehicles to store the equipment that is used to initiate cooling, lack of credentialing for the use of paralytic agents, and difficulty in prioritizing for training and patient care.[76] Another problem noted from some of the clinical studies addressed above is that after induction of hypothermia in the field, some patients were transported to hospitals where TH is not systematically continued in the post resuscitation care occurring in-hospital. If a patient is cooled only to be rewarmed soon after transport to a facilty, then this may actually be worse than not cooling the patient to begin with, as this might reverse and maybe even cause a rebound in all of the mechanisms of secondary injury (ischemia-reperfusion) discussed above. Hence, it is very important that these patients be transported to a facilty staffed and equipped with the ability to continue inhospital therapeutic hypothermia for at least 12-24 hours in addition to the other bundles of resuscitative care.[7]

7. Conclusion

Animal and laboratory data have suggested that there is significantly decreased neurological injury if cooling is initiated as soon as possible after resuscitation. Human clinical studies are either underpowered or due to study design do not allow conclusions regarding effects on outcome to be drawn, but the safety and feasibility of early cooling was strongly demonstrated. Prehospital cooling comes with its own logistic challenges, such as limitation of EMS vehicle space, lack of ideal equipment for induction of hypothermia and for temperature monitoring, lack of credentialing for use of paralytic agents by EMS teams that are not staffed by physicians, transport to facilities that are not equipped to continue inhospital therapeutic hypothermia and postresuscitation care, the potential for overcooling and shivering, and interference with basic resuscitation efforts in the field. Intraarest and postarrest bundles of care that include therapeutic hypothermia, as well as training of EMS teams, EMS physicians, emergency room staff, cardiologists and cardiac catheterization lab staff, and intensive care unit physicians and staff on these protocols and bundles are crucial for the success of these bundles and the implementation of this important therapy, whether cooling is initiated in the field or in the hospital setting. Clearly, large prospective randomized controlled trials of prehospital therapeutic hypothermia preferably as part of a cardiac arrest bundle of care are needed.

Author details

Farid Sadaka

Mercy Hospital St Louis/St Louis University, Critical Care Medicine/Neurocritical Care, St Louis, USA

Acknowledgement

No additional acknowledgements.

Conflicts of Interest

The author reports no conflicts of interest.

The author declares that No competing financial interests exist.

The author reports that no potential conflicts of interest exist with any companies/organizations whose products or services may be discussed in this article.

8. References

[1] Stiell IG, Wells GA, Field B, Spaite DW, Nesbitt LP, De Maio VJ, Nichol G, Cousineau D, Blackburn J, Munkley D, Luinstra-Toohey L, Campeau T, Dagnone E, Lyver M; Ontario Prehospital Advanced Life Support Study Group (2004) Advanced cardiac life support in out-of-hospital cardiac arrest. N Engl J Med 351:647– 656.

[2] Keenan SP, Dodek P, Martin C, Priestap F, Norena M, Wong H (2007) Variation in length of intensive care unit stay after cardiac arrest: where you are is as important as who you are. Crit Care Med 35: 836–841.

[3] Mashiko K, Otsuka T, Shimazaki S, Kohama A, Kamishima G, Katsurada K, Sawada Y, Matsubara I, Yamaguchi K (2002) An outcome study of out-of-hospital cardiac arrest using the Utstein template: a Japanese experience. Resuscitation 55:241–246.

[4] Nolan JP, Laver SR, Welch CA, Harrison DA, Gupta V, Rowan K (2007) Outcome following admission to UK intensive care units after cardiac arrest: a secondary analysis of the ICNARC Case Mix Programme Database. Anaesthesia 62:1207–1216.

[5] Langhelle A, Tyvold SS, Lexow K, Hapnes SA, Sunde K, Steen PA (2003) In-hospital factors associated with improved outcome after out-ofhospital cardiac arrest: a comparison between four regions in Norway. Resuscitation 56:247–263.

[6] Herlitz J, Engdahl J, Svensson L, Angquist KA, Silfverstolpe J, Holmberg S (2006) Major differences in 1-month survival between hospitals in Sweden among initial survivors of out-of-hospital cardiac arrest. Resuscitation 70:404–409.

[7] Neumar RW, Nolan JP, Adrie C, Aibiki M, Berg RA, Böttiger BW, Callaway C, Clark RSB, Geocadin RG, Jauch EC, Kern KB, Laurent I, Longstreth WT Jr, Merchant RM, Morley P, Morrison LJ, Nadkarni V, Peberdy MA, Rivers EP, Rodriguez-Nunez A, Sellke FW, Spaulding C, Sunde K, Vanden Hoek T (2008) Post– cardiac arrest syndrome: epidemiology, pathophysiology, treatment, and prognostication: a consensus statement from the International Liaison Committee on Resuscitation (American Heart Association, Australian and New Zealand Council on Resuscitation, European Resuscitation Council, Heart and Stroke Foundation of Canada, InterAmerican Heart Foundation, Resuscitation Council of Asia, and the Resuscitation Council of Southern Africa); the American Heart Association Emergency Cardiovascular Care Committee; the Council on Cardiovascular Surgery and Anesthesia; the Council on Cardiopulmonary, Perioperative, and Critical Care; the Council on Clinical Cardiology; and the Stroke Council. Circulation 118:2452–2483.

[8] Eisenberg MS, Mengert TJ (2001) Cardiac Resuscitation. N Engl J Med 334: 1304-1313.

[9] Bunch TJ, White RD, Smith GE, Hodge DO, Gersh BJ, Hammill SC, Shen WK, Packer DL (1998) Long-term subjective memory function in ventricular fibrillation out-of-hospital cardiac arrest survivors resuscitated by early defibrillation. Resuscitation 36:111-122.

[10] Laver S, Farrow C, Turner D, Nolan J (2004) Mode of death after admission to an intensive care unit following cardiac arrest. Intensive Care Med 30:2126 –2128.

[11] Jacobs I, Nadkarni V, Bahr J, Berg RA, Billi JE, Bossaert L, Cassan P, Coovadia A, D'Este K, Finn J, Halperin H, Handley A, Herlitz J, Hickey R, Idris A, Kloeck W, Larkin GL, Mancini ME, Mason P, Mears G, Monsieurs K, Montgomery W, Morley P, Nichol G, Nolan J, Okada K, Perlman J, Shuster M, Steen PA, Sterz F, Tibballs J, Timerman S, Truitt T, Zideman D; International Liaison Committee on Resuscitation (2004) Cardiac arrest and cardiopulmonary resuscitation outcome reports: update and simplification of the Utstein templates for resuscitation registries: a statement for healthcare professionals from a task force of the International Liaison Committee on Resuscitation (American Heart Association, European Resuscitation Council, Australian Resuscitation Council, New Zealand Resuscitation Council, Heart and Stroke Foundation of Canada, InterAmerican Heart Foundation, Resuscitation Council of Southern Africa). Resuscitation 63:233–249.

[12] Hypothermia After Cardiac Arrest Study Group (2002) Mild therapeutic hypothermia to improve the neurologic outcome after cardiac arrest. N Engl J Med 346:549 –556.

[13] Bernard SA, Gray TW, Buist MD, Jones BM, Silvester W, Gutteridge G, Smith K (2002) Treatment of comatose survivors of out-of-hospital cardiac arrest with induced hypothermia. N Engl J Med 346:557–563.

[14] Holzer M, Bernard SA, Hachimi-Idrissi S, Roine RO, Sterz F, Müllner M; Collaborative Group on Induced Hypothermia for Neuroprotection After Cardiac Arrest (2005) Hypothermia for neuroprotection after cardiac arrest: systematic review and individual patient data meta-analysis. Crit Care Med 33:414–418.

[15] Oddo M, Schaller MD, Feihl F, Ribordy V, Liaudet L (2006) From evidence to clinical practice: effective implementation of therapeutic hypothermia to improve patient outcome after cardiac arrest. Crit Care Med 34: 1865–1873.

[16] Sunde K, Pytte M, Jacobsen D, Mangschau A, Jensen LP, Smedsrud C, Draegni T, Steen PA (2007) Implementation of a standardised treatment protocol for post resuscitation care after out-of-hospital cardiac arrest. Resuscitation 73:29 –39.

[17] Busch M, Soreide E, Lossius HM, Lexow K, Dickstein K (2006) Rapid implementation of therapeutic hypothermia in comatose out-of-hospital cardiac arrest survivors. Acta Anaesthesiol Scand 50:1277–1283.

[18] Arrich J; European Resuscitation Council Hypothermia After Cardiac Arrest Registry Study Group (2007) Clinical application of mild therapeutic hypothermia after cardiac arrest. Crit Care Med 35:1041–1047.

[19] Holzer M, Müllner M, Sterz F, Robak O, Kliegel A, Losert H, Sodeck G, Uray T, Zeiner A, Laggner AN (2006) Efficacy and safety of endovascular cooling after cardiac arrest: cohort study and Bayesian approach. Stroke 37:1792–1797.

[20] 2005 American Heart Association Guidelines for Cardiopulmonary Resuscitation and Emergency Cardiovascular Care Part 7.5: Postresuscitation Support. Circulation 112:IV-84–IV- 88.

[21] Peberdy MA, Callaway CW, Neumar RW, Geocadin RG, Zimmerman JL, Donnino M, Gabrielli A, Silvers SM, Zaritsky AL, Merchant R, Vanden Hoek TL, Kronick SL (2010) Part 9: post- cardiac arrest care: 2010 American Heart Association Guidelines for Cardiopulmonary Resuscitation and Emergency Cardiovascular Care. Circulation 122 (suppl 3):S768 –S786.

[22] Polderman KH (2008) Induced hypothermia and fever control for prevention and treatment of neurological injuries. Lancet 371: 1955–1969.

[23] Small DL, Morley P, Buchan AM (1999) Biology of ischemic cerebral cell death. Prog Cardiovasc Dis 42:185–207.

[24] Hagerdal M, Harp J, Nilsson L, Siesjö BK (1975) The effect of induced hypothermia upon oxygen consumption in the rat brain. J Neurochem 24:311–316.

[25] Povlishock JT, Buki A, Koiziumi H, Stone J, Okonkwo DO (1999) Initiating mechanisms involved in the pathobiology of traumatically induced axonal injury and interventions targeted at blunting their progression. Acta Neurochir Suppl (Wien) 73:15–20

[26] Xu L, Yenari MA, Steinberg GK, Giffard RG (2002) Mild hypothermia reduces apoptosis of mouse neurons in vitro early in the cascade. J Cereb Blood Flow Metab 22:21–28

[27] Ning XH, Chen SH, Xu CS, Li L, Yao LY, Qian K, Krueger JJ, Hyyti OM, Portman MA (2002) Hypothermic protection of the ischemic heart via alterations in apoptotic pathways as assessed by gene array analysis. J Appl Physiol 92:2200–2207

[28] Siesjo BK, Bengtsson F, Grampp W, Theander S (1989) Calcium, excitotoxins, and neuronal death in brain. Ann NY Acad Sci 568: 234–251.

[29] Leker RR, Shohami E (2002) Cerebral ischemia and trauma—different etiologies yet similar mechanisms: Neuroprotective opportunities. Brain Res Brain Res Rev 39: 55–73

[30] Dempsey RJ, Combs DJ, Maley ME, Cowen DE, Roy MW, Donaldson DL (1987) Moderate hypothermia reduces postischemic edema development and leukotriene production. Neurosurgery 21:177–181.

[31] Globus MY-T, Alonso O, Dietrich WD, Busto R, Ginsberg MD (1995) Glutamate release and free radical production following brain injury: Effects of posttraumatic hypothermia. J Neurochem 65:1704–1711.

[32] Busto R, Globus MY, Dietrich WD, Martinez E, Valdés I, Ginsberg MD (1989) Effect of mild hypothermia on ischemia-induced release of neurotransmitters and free fatty acids in rat brain. Stroke 20:904–910.

[33] Takata K, Takeda Y, Morita K (2005) Effects of hypothermia for a short period on histological outcome and extracellular glutamate concentration during and after cardiac arrest in rats. Crit Care Med 33: 1340–1345.

[34] Kuboyama K, Safar P, Radovsky A, Tisherman SA, Stezoski SW, Alexander H (1993) Delay in cooling negates the beneficial effect of mild resuscitative cerebral hypothermia after cardiac arrest in dogs: A prospective, randomized study. Crit Care Med 21:1348–1358.

[35] Aibiki M, Maekawa S, Ogura S, Kinoshita Y, Kawai N, Yokono S (1999) Effect of moderate hypothermia on systemic and internal jugular plasma IL-6 levels after traumatic brain injury in humans. J Neurotrauma 16:225–232.

[36] Schmidt OI, Heyde CE, Ertel W, Stahel PF (2005) Closed head injury—an inflammatory disease? Brain Res Brain Res Rev 48: 388–399.

[37] Kimura A, Sakurada S, Ohkuni H, Todome Y, Kurata K (2002) Moderate hypothermia delays proinflammatory cytokine production of human peripheral blood mononuclear cells. Crit Care Med 30:1499–1502.

[38] Dietrich WD, Chatzipanteli K, Vitarbo E, Wada K, Kinoshita K (2004) The role of inflammatory processes in the pathophysiology and treatment of brain and spinal cord trauma. Acta Neurochir Suppl 89:69–74.

[39] Chi OZ, Liu X, Weiss HR (2001) Effects of mild hypothermia on blood– brain barrier disruption during isoflurane or pentobarbital anesthesia. Anesthesiology 95:933–938.

[40] Smith SL, Hall ED (1996) Mild pre- and posttraumatic hypothermia attenuates blood–brain barrier damage following controlled cortical impact injury in the rat. J Neurotrauma 13:1–9.

[41] Jurkovich GJ, Pitt RM, Curreri PW, Granger DN (1988) Hypothermia prevents increased capillary permeability following ischemia–reperfusion injury. J Surg Res 44:514–521.

[42] Bo¨ttiger BW, Motsch J, Bohrer H, Böker T, Aulmann M, Nawroth PP, Martin E (1995) Activation of blood coagulation after cardiac arrest is not balanced adequately by activation of endogenous fibrinolysis. Circulation 92:2572–2578.

[43] Gando S, Kameue T, Nanzaki S, Nakanishi Y (1997) Massive fibrin formation with consecutive impairment of fibrinolysis in patients with out-of-hospital cardiac arrest. Thromb Haemost 77:278–282.

[44] Michelson AD, MacGregor H, Barnard MR, Kestin AS, Rohrer MJ, Valeri CR (1994) Hypothermia-induced reversible platelet dysfunction. Thromb Haemost 71:633–640.

[45] Valeri CR, MacGregor H, Cassidy G, Tinney R, Pompei F (1995) Effects of temperature on bleeding time and clotting time in normal male and female volunteers. Crit Care Med 23: 698–704.

[46] Chen ST, Hsu CY, Hogan EL, Halushka PV, Linet OI, Yatsu FM (1986) Thromboxane, prostacyclin, and leukotrienes in cerebral ischemia. Neurology 36: 466–470.

[47] Maekawa S, Aibiki M, Ogura S (1997) Mild hypothermia suppresses thromboxane B2 production in brain-injured patients. In: The Immune Consequences of Trauma, Shock and Sepsis. Mechanisms and Therapeutic Approaches. Faist E (Ed). Bologna, Italy, Monduzzi Editore pp 135–138.

[48] Aibiki M, Maekawa S, Yokono S (2000) Moderate hypothermia improves imbalances of thromboxane A2 and prostaglandin I2 production after traumatic brain injury in humans. Crit Care Med 28:3902–3906.

[49] Kuboyama K, Safar P, Radovsky A, Tisherman SA, Stezoski SW, Alexander H (1993) Delay in cooling negates the beneficial effect of mild resuscitative cerebral hypothermia after cardiac arrest in dogs: a prospective, randomized study. Crit Care Med 21:1348 – 1358.

[50] Abella BS, Zhao D, Alvarado J, Hamann K, Vanden Hoek TL, Becker LB (2004) Intra-arrest cooling improves outcomes in a murine cardiac arrest model. Circulation 109:2786 –2791.

[51] Colbourne F, Sutherland GR, Auer RN (1999) Electron microscopic evidence against apoptosis as the mechanism of neuronal death in global ischemia. J Neurosci 19:4200–4210.

[52] Zhao D, Abella BS, Beiser DG, Alvarado JP, Wang H, Hamann KJ, Hoek TL, Becker LB (2008) Intra-arrest cooling with delayed reperfusion yields higher survival than earlier normothermic resuscitation in a mouse model of cardiac arrest. Resuscitation 77:242–249.

[53] Nozari A, Safar P, Stezoski SW, Wu X, Kostelnik S, Radovsky A, Tisherman S, Kochanek PM (2006) Critical time window for intraarrest cooling with cold saline flush in a dog model of cardiopulmonary resuscitation. Circulation 113:2690–2696.

[54] Bernard S, Buist M, Monteiro O, Smith K (2003) Induced hypothermia using large volume, ice-cold intravenous fluid in comatose survivors of out-of- hospital cardiac arrest: a preliminary report. Resuscitation 56:9 –13.

[55] Polderman KH, Rijnsburger ER, Peerdeman SM, Girbes AR (2005) Induction of hypothermia in patients with various types of neurologic injury with use of large volumes of ice-cold intravenous fluid. Crit Care Med 33:2744 –2751.

[56] Kim F, Olsufka M, Longstreth WT Jr, Maynard C, Carlbom D, Deem S, Kudenchuk P, Copass MK, Cobb LA (2007) Pilot randomized clinical trial of prehospital induction of mild hypothermia in out ofhospital cardiac arrest patients with a rapid infusion of 4 degrees C normal saline. Circulation 115:3064-70.

[57] Kämäräinen A, Virkkunen I, Tenhunen J, Yli-Hankala A, Silfvast T (2009) Prehospital therapeutic hypothermia for comatose survivors of cardiac arrest: a randomized controlled trial. Acta Anaesthesiol Scand 53:900-7.

[58] Bernard SA, Smith K, Cameron P, Masci K, Taylor DM, Cooper DJ, Kelly AM, Silvester W; Rapid Infusion of Cold Hartmanns (RICH) Investigators (2010) Induction of therapeutic hypothermia by paramedics after resuscitation from out-of-hospital ventricular fibrillation cardiac arrest: a randomized controlled trial. Circulation 122(7):737-42.

[59] Bernard SA, Smith K, Cameron P, Masci K, Taylor DM, Cooper DJ, Kelly AM, Silvester W; Rapid Infusion of Cold Hartmanns (RICH) Investigators (2012) Induction of prehospital therapeutic hypothermia after resuscitation from nonventricular fibrillation cardiac arrest. Crit Care Med 40(3):747-53.

[60] Castre´n M, Nordberg P, Svensson L, Taccone F, Vincent JL, Desruelles D, Eichwede F, Mols P, Schwab T, Vergnion M, Storm C, Pesenti A, Pachl J, Gue´risse F, Elste T, Roessler M, Fritz H, Durnez P, Busch H-J, Inderbitzen B, Barbut D (2010) Intra-arrest transnasal evaporative cooling: a randomized, prehospital, multicenter study (PRINCE: Pre-ROSC Intra-Nasal Cooling Effectiveness). Circulation 122:729–736.

[61] Callaway C, Tadler S, Katz L, Lipinski C, Brader E (2002) Feasibility of external cranial cooling during out-of-hospital cardiac arrest. Resuscitation 52:159-65.

[62] Virkkunen I, Yli-Hankala A, Silfvast T (2004) Induction of therapeutic hypothermia after cardiac arrest in prehospital patients using ice-cold Ringer's solution: a pilot study. Resuscitation. 62:299-302.

[63] Uray T, Malzer R, on behalf of the Vienna Hypothermia After Cardiac Arrest (HACA) Study Group (2008) Out-of-hospital surface cooling to induce mild hypothermia in human cardiac arrest: A feasibility trial. Resuscitation 77:331-338.

[64] Hammer L, Vitrat F, Savary D, Debaty G, Santre C, Durand M, Dessertaine G, Timsit JF (2009) Immediate prehospital hypothermia protocol in comatose survivors of out-of-hospital cardiac arrest. Am J Emerg Med. 27:570-3.

[65] Storm C, Schefold JC, Kerner T, Schmidbauer W, Gloza J, Krueger A, Jörres A, Hasper D (2008) Prehospital cooling with hypothermia caps (PreCoCa): a feasibility study. Clin Res Cardiol 97:768-72.

[66] Kämäräinen A, Virkkunen I, Tenhunen J, Yli-Hankala A, Silfvast T (2008) Induction of therapeutic hypothermia during prehospital CPR using ice-cold intravenous fluid. Resuscitation 79:205-11.

[67] Bruel C, Parienti JJ, Marie W, Arrot X, Daubin C, Du Cheyron D, Massetti M, Charbonneau P (2008) Mild hypothermia during advanced life support: a preliminary study in out-of-hospital cardiac arrest. Crit Care 12:R31.

[68] Garrett JS, Studnek JR, Blackwell T, Vandeventer S, Pearson DA, Heffner AC, Reades R (2011) The association between intra-arrest therapeutic hypothermia and return of

spontaneous circulation among individuals experiencing out of hospital cardiac arrest. Resuscitation 82(1):21-5.

[69] Mader TJ (2009) The effect of ambient temperature on cold saline during simulated infusion to induce therapeutic hypothermia. Resuscitation 80:766–768.

[70] Spaite DW, Bobrow BJ, Vadeboncoeur TF, Chikani V, Clark L, Mullins T, Sanders AB (2008) The impact of prehospital transport interval on survival in out-of-hospital cardiac arrest: implications for regionalization of post-resuscitation care. Resuscitation 79:61–66.

[71] Riter HG, Brooks LA, Pretorius AM, Ackermann LW, Kerber RE (2009) Intra-arrest hypothermia: both cold liquid ventilation with perfluorocarbons and cold intravenous saline rapidly achieve hypothermia, but only cold liquid ventilation improves resumption of spontaneous circulation. Resuscitation 80: 561–566.

[72] Laven BA, Kasza KE, Rapp DE, Orvieto MA, Lyon MB, Oras JJ, Beiser DG, Vanden Hoek TL, Son H, Shalhav AL (2007) A pilot study of ice-slurry application for inducing laparoscopic renal hypothermia. BJU Int 99:166–170.

[73] Weinrauch V, Safar P, Tisherman S, Kuboyama K, Radovsky A (1992) Beneficial effect of mild hypothermia and detrimental effect of deep hypothermia after cardiac arrest in dogs. Stroke 23:1454–1462.

[74] Sessler DI (2001 Complications and treatment of mild hypothermia. Anesthesiology 95: 531–543.

[75] Merchant RM, Abella BS, Peberdy MA, Soar J, Ong ME, Schmidt GA, Becker LB, Vanden Hoek TL (2006) Therapeutic hypothermia after cardiac arrest: unintentional overcooling is common using ice packs and conventional cooling blankets. Crit Care Med 34:S490–S494.

[76] Suffoletto BP, Salcido DD, Menegazzi JJ (2008) Use of prehospitalinduced hypothermia after out-of-hospital cardiac arrest: a survey of the National Association of Emergency Medical Services Physicians. Prehosp Emerg Care 12:52–56.

Section 3

Therapeutic Hypothermia-Stroke / SCI

Chapter 4

Therapeutic Hypothermia in Acute Stroke

Edgar A. Samaniego

Additional information is available at the end of the chapter

http://dx.doi.org/10.5772/51071

1. Introduction

Stroke is the second most common cause of death and a major cause of serious long-term disability in adults in industrialized countries. Approximately 90% of strokes are ischemic and the rest are hemorrhagic.[1] Unfortunately, few effective treatments can be offered during the acute and subacute phases. Since the introduction of tissue plasminogen activator (tPA) in 1995, there are no other medical treatments for ischemic stroke besides the use of antiplatelets for primary and secondary prevention. Moreover, the clinical treatments for hemorrhagic stroke are also limited.

In ischemic stroke most of therapies aim to recanalize the vessel and restore flow through pharmacological or endovascular treatments. However, another approach to preserve brain tissue is through the interruption of catalytic pathways triggered by ischemia. Rapid restoration of oxygen and glucose by thrombolysis will always provide the most effective neuroprotection, but directly targeting the brain parenchyma to confer neuroprotection may be a viable alternative, particularly in conjunction with thrombolysis. Multiple pharmacological attempts have failed in finding an ideal neuroprotective agent. Over 1000 neuroprotective agents have been tested in basic stroke studies with many showing promise.[2] However, to date no neuroprotective agent has successfully transitioned from bench or animal studies into clinical use. Although cooling may be unable to salvage neural tissue that has irreversibly progressed to infarction, hypothermia minimizes the extent of secondary injury as an acute or subacute treatment strategy. Hypothermia is increasingly being used, especially since therapeutic mild hypothermia has demonstrated to positively influence neurological outcome in humans following acute brain injuries, namely, global ischemic brain injury due to cardiac arrest and hypoxic-ischemic encephalopathy in neonates.[3, 4]

Catalytic cascades are generated in the brain tissue surrounding a blood clot after intracerebral hemorrhage (ICH). Hypothermia may also be used as a neuroprotection treatment in these circumstances. Hypothermia has the potential to minimize secondary injury resulting from insufficient cerebral perfusion pressure or mechanical compression from herniation by ICH. Hypothermia preserves autoregulation of the cerebral vasculature and reduces cytotoxic edema around the hemorrhagic clot.[5]

2. Pathophysiology of ischemic brain injury

Ischemic brain injury is composed by the initial ischemic cascade and reperfusion injury.[6] During cerebral ischemia, cessation of blood flow and hypoxia trigger a complex set of metabolic and biochemical processes that comprise the ischemic cascade. An initial event in the ischemic cascade is the depletion of adenosine triphosphate (ATP), which is generated by oxygen-dependent phosphorylation in the central nervous system. ATP depletion leads to neurolemma depolarization secondary to derangement of Na^+ and K^+ gradients and, consequently, inappropriate accumulation of intracellular Ca^{2+} resulting from both Ca^{2+} influx and release from intracellular Ca^{2+} stores.[7] Increased intracellular Ca^{2+} concentration causes promiscuous activation of multiple intracellular enzyme systems, including protein kinase C, protein kinase B, calcium/calmodulin-dependent protein kinase II, mitogen-activated protein kinases, and phospholipases A_2, C, and D. Prolonged elevations in intracellular Ca^{2+} concentration trigger the release of neurotrasmitters, which couples with the activation of multiple enzyme systems, inevitably leading to necrotic cell death through membrane dissolution if ischemia continues. In dogs, when ischemic brain is reperfused within 3 to 12 minutes, neuronal ATP production appears to recover rapidly, with replenishment of baseline cellular levels within 6 minutes.[8] However, after 30 minutes of ischemia, the replenishment of ATP to baseline levels takes significantly longer (~36 minutes).[9] Furthermore, even after 3 hours of reperfusion after intracranial thrombus injection, brain ATP levels still may not return to baseline levels.[10] Therefore, timely reperfusion is paramount, and after reperfusion is established, the direct cytotoxic effects of the ischemic cascade likely continue for minutes to hours until cellular ATP levels recover sufficiently.

3. Hypothermia at the cellular level

Hypothermia is neuroprotective through several mechanisms. The effects of hypothermia include a wide range of biological processes which include decreasing excitatory amino acid release, reducing free radical formation, enhancing small ubiquitin-related modifier-related pathways, attenuating protein kinase C activity and slowing cellular metabolism.[11-13] Hypothermia has little effect on the core of infarcted tissue, but acts on tissue at risk in the penumbra by modulating different mechanisms that lead to cellular injury and death.[14] A marked reduction in the metabolic demand of penumbral tissue with induced hypothermia may prevent damage due to oxidative stress and energy failure. Cooling also results in reduced proteolysis and excitotoxic damage caused by glutamate toxicity, and reduction in neuronal calcium influx.[15, 16]

For every 1 °C reduction in brain temperature, the cerebral metabolic rate decreases in 6%. [17] Under stress conditions, hypothermia decreases high energy organic phosphates losses, slows the rates of metabolite consumption and lactic acid accumulation and reduces cerebral metabolic oxygen consumption, while improving glucose utilization.[11]

Hypothermia not only protects the brain by reducing cerebral metabolism during conditions of reduced substrate and shift to anaerobic glycolysis. Hypothermia also suppresses the accumulation and release of glutamate.[18] ATP loss during ischemia leads to ions flowing down their concentration gradients, and eventual efflux of potassium and influx of sodium and calcium.[19] Calcium influxes lead to direct neurotoxicity as well as extracellular accumulation of glutamate, which are neurotoxic. Experimental studies have shown that mild to moderate hypothermia attenuates the initial and delayed rise of extracellular potassium and prevents intracellular calcium accumulation, thus leading to decreased glutamate efflux and finally neuroprotection.

Numerous studies have shown that hypothermia reduces the generation of reactive oxygen species, decreases brain edema, and prevents blood-brain barrier breakdown.[18] One potential mechanism is that hypothermia inhibits matrix metalloproteinases and preserves basal lamina proteins after stroke.[20-22] Moreover, a clinical study of 10 patients with large strokes who underwent mild hypothermia demonstrated lower levels of matrix metalloproteinase than normothermic patients.[23] Serum metalloproteinases are a good marker of blood-brain barrier breakdown.[20]

Hypothermia has been documented by numerous investigators to alter gene expression normally observed after brain ischemia. Whereas a majority of genes are downregulated by hypothermia, a number of genes are also upregulated. [24] Interestingly, many proinflammatory and proapoptotic genes tend to be downregulated.[25-27] Whereas those genes that contribute to cell survival seem to be upregulated. [28-32]

Additionally, hypothermia has been shown to inhibit activation of the inflammatory transcription factor nuclear factor kappa B via temperature-dependent inhibition of its inhibitor protein's kinase. Other studies indicate that hypothermia has antiapoptotic effects such as reduction of cytochrome C release, and inhibition of caspases and proapoptotic genes.[33-37]

4. Cooling temperatures

Therapeutic hypothermia is defined as an intentionally induced, controlled reduction of a patient's core temperature below 36°C. Further classification includes mild (34°C–35.9°C), moderate (32°C–33.9°C), moderate/deep (30°C–31.9°C), and deep (< 30°C) hypothermia. [38]

In general, hypothermia appears to be effective whether the brain is cooled to 33°C or 28°C, but temperatures on the lower end appeared to be most effective according to a recent meta-analysis of the experimental literature.[39] However, lower temperatures are associated with a higher incidence of complications, require more sedation and sometimes even induction of paralysis accompanied by intubation and ventilatory support.

5. Hypothermia in ischemic stroke

Body temperature is increased in 4% to 25 % of patients with acute ischemic stroke within the first six hours after symptom onset.[40] The pathophysiology of this increase in body temperature is not completely understood. Higher body temperature may be a natural consequence of brain infarction. However, animal studies have suggested that higher body temperatures may increase the damage induced by cerebral ischemia.[41] Observational studies in patients with acute stroke have established the influence of body temperature on the clinical outcome of stroke. For each 1 °C increase in body temperature, the relative risk of poor outcome worsens more than two times.[42] This association may be limited to the first 12 to 24 hours from stroke onset.[42] These studies therefore suggest that control of body temperature and fever prevention may improve functional outcome after stroke.

In a systematic review of animal studies, therapeutic hypothermia reduced infarct size by 44% (95% confidence interval 40 to 47%). The best results were obtained with lower temperatures (≤ 31 °C), when treatment was started before or at the onset of ischemia, and in temporary rather than permanent ischemia models. However, a reduction in infarct volume by about one third was also observed with temperature reduction to 35 °C, with initiation of treatment between 90 and 180 minutes, and in permanent ischemia models.[39] The effects of hypothermia on functional outcome were broadly similar.[39] This suggests that temperature-lowering therapy might be effective for large numbers of patients with ischemic stroke.

6. Human studies of hypothermia in ischemic stroke

Clinical studies of induced hypothermia were conducted on humans based on successful cerebral ischemia animal models. One of the first studies cooled 17 patients with stroke admitted within 12 hours from symptom onset (mean 3.25 hours) for 6 hours.[43] Hypothermia was induced (35.5° C) with cooling blankets and shivering was treated with meperidine. Mortality at 6 months after stroke was 12% in the hypothermia group versus 23% in historical matched-controls. Unfortunately, no benefit in terms of outcome was observed. It has been suggested that a longer hypothermia duration of 48–72 h may be required to reduce the formation of cerebral edema which usually occurs during the first 72-h after symptom onset.

Another study by Keller and collaborators measured the cerebral blood flow (CBF) and cerebral metabolic rate of oxygen consumption ($CMRO_2$) in six patients with middle cerebral artery (MCA) strokes treated with hypothermia.[44] Patients were intubated and cooled with cooling blankets for 48 to 96 hours. A total of 19 measurements of CBF and jugular bulb O_2 saturation were performed. This preliminary study suggested that moderate hypothermia (33° C) seems to reduce CBF and $CMRO_2$ in humans.

A small study evaluated the feasibility of inducing and maintaining moderate hypothermia with the use of endovascular rather than surface cooling.[45] Six patients with severe acute ischemic stroke were treated with moderate hypothermia. The pace of cooling was 1.4 +/-

0.6º C/h, and target temperature was reached after 3 +/- 1 h (range, 2 to 4.5 h). During hypothermia, the maximal temperature observed was 33.4º C, and the minimal temperature was 32.2º C. Every patient developed pneumonia and hypotension. This small study demonstrated that induction and maintenance of hypothermia with an intravenous cooling device was feasible.

Cooling for acute ischemic brain damage (COOL-AID), was one of the first studies to evaluate hypothermia in ischemic stroke after thrombolysis.[46] This was a nonrandomized study that used surface cooling to achieve a cooling temperature of 32 ± 1°C for 12 to 72-h. To prevent shivering, all patients undergoing hypothermia were intubated, sedated, and pharmacologically paralyzed. The study demonstrated that hypothermia is technically feasible and safe for patients with acute ischemic strokes who are undergoing thrombolytic therapy. However, the study was too small (10 patients) to determine any solid conclusions.

A later version of the same study, evaluated and intravascular cooling device in the treatment of stroke through the induction of hypothermia. The second COOL-AID was a randomized controlled study of 40 patients presenting within 12- h of symptom onset. Eighteen patients were cooled and 22 received standard medical management, which included thrombolysis in 13 patients. Shivering was suppressed using a forced-air warming blanket, buspirone and meperidine. Eight patients in the hypothermia group required intubation during their hospitalization, one patient was intubated during the maintenance phase of hypothermia and the other for various reasons not related to cooling. Most patients tolerated hypothermia, and clinical outcomes were similar in both groups although there was a trend of reduced lesion growth on diffusion-weighted imaging in the group treated with hypothermia.[47] Side effects included pneumonia, cardiac arrhythmia, and deep vein thrombosis. The main lessons from these two studies (COOL-AID one and two) were that mild hypothermia can be achieved in awake patients with the appropriate cooling and anti-shivering protocols; and that endovascular cooling achieves target temperature faster than surface cooling.

ICTuS is another nonrandomized clinical trial that cooled 18 acute stroke patients using an endovascular cooling device.[48] Patients were cooled within 12 hours of symptom onset. An anti-shivering regimen with buspirone and meperidine was administered prophylactically. Overall, patients tolerated cooling well and the incidence of cerebral hemorrhage did not increase among patients (n=5) who received intravenous (IV) tPA. This trial confirmed that endovascular cooling with a proactive anti-shivering regimen can be accomplished in awake stroke patients. A later brain CT analysis of patients who were effectively cooled (n=7) versus those who were not (n=11), suggested that endovascular hypothermia decreases acute post-ichemic cerebral edema. [49] At the end of the cooling and rewarming period (36–48 h), patients who were effectively cooled had significantly decreased cerebral edema compared to patients who were either ineffectively cooled or not cooled at all. The effect disappeared by 30 days, as might be expected given the natural course of post-infarction cerebral edema.

A follow-up randomized, controlled study of endovascular cooling in awake patients after stroke (ICTuS-L), studied hypothermia with thrombolysis in patients presenting with acute ischemic stroke < 6 h from symptom onset.[50] Twenty eight patients were randomized to receive hypothermia and 30 to normothermia. There were no differences in outcome or incidence of adverse events comparing patients who were treated with tPA and hypothermia with those who were not cooled. For safety concerns, endovascular hypothermia with placement of the femoral cooling catheter was not begun until 30 to 180 minutes after completion of the tPA infusion, delaying cooling. Pneumonia was more frequent after hypothermia, although the occurrence of pneumonia did not significantly affect outcome at 90 days. The study used meperidine, oral buspirone, and surface skin warming to prevent shivering in awake patients. This study demonstrated the feasibility and preliminary safety of combining endovascular hypothermia after stroke with intravenous thrombolysis, similarly to what the COOL AID study demonstrated previously.[46]

The experience in the use of hypothermia with thrombolysis is limited in stroke patients. In the first COOL-AID study that used surface cooling, 4 of 10 patients received intra-arterial thrombolysis, and 2 received IV therapy.[46] In the second study, 3 of 18 patients were treated with intra-arterial therapy, and 10 received IV thrombolysis.[47] One patient who was treated with hypothermia and intra-arterial thrombolysis experienced retroperitoneal hemorrhage.[47] In the ICTuS-L trial, the rate of ICH was similar among patients who received tPA with hypothermia and those treated with tPA alone.[51]

Hypothermia has also been studied with other neuroprotective agents in the treatment of acute ischemic stroke. Twenty patients with acute ischemic stroke were treated with caffeinol (caffeine 8-9 mg/kg + ethanol 0.4 g/kg intravenously x 2 hours, started by 4 hours after symptom onset) and hypothermia (started by 5 hours and continued for 24 hours (33-35º C), followed by 12 hours of rewarming).[52] IV tPA was given to 16 patients within 3 hours of symptom onset. Meperidine and buspirone were used to suppress shivering. Cooling was successfully achieved in 16 patients via endovascular and surface approaches. All patients reached target temperature, on average within 2 hours and 30 minutes from induction and 6 hours and 21 minutes from symptom onset. Three patients died: one from symptomatic hemorrhage, one from malignant cerebral edema, and one from unrelated medical complications. No adverse events were attributed to caffeinol.

A small study evaluated the use of ice-cold saline for the induction of mild hypothermia in 10 patients with acute ischemic stroke.[53] Ice-cold saline at 4°C (25 mL/kg body weight) was administered one time to induce mild hypothermia. Patients received buspirone and meperidine to prevent and treat shivering. Tympanic temperature dropped significantly by a maximum of 1.6 ± 0.3°C at 52 ± 16 minutes after ice-cold saline was started. The procedure was well tolerated, however, hypothermia was not maintained after the infusion of ice-cold saline.

7. Hypothermia and thrombolysis

Theoretically, the combination of hypothermia with pharmacological thrombolysis to restore blood flow and provide neuroprotection is a very promising strategy. However, many serine proteases are affected by temperature, and the activity of tPA may be reduced in hypothermia.[54] In vitro analysis shows that cooling to 30°C to 33°C decreases tPA activity by 2% to 4%.[55] Moreover, it has been reported that the response to tPA may be related to body temperature at stroke presentation.[56] Investigators studied 111 acute stroke patients given tPA and found that patients presenting with a higher body temperature were more likely to have a favorable outcome compared with patients presenting with lower body temperatures. The authors suggested that this surprising finding might be explained by the benefit of im proved clot lysis by tPA at higher temperatures compared with the potential neuroprotective benefit of lower body temperature.

A recent analysis of 5586 patients with acute ischemic stroke (1980 patients received tPA) determined that tPA treatment effect was not associated with baseline temperature.[57] Point estimates showed benefit of tPA treatment across 35.5°C to 37.5°C but showed a negative trend >37.5°C. Temperature profiles did not influence tPA effectiveness over 72 hours after stroke.

8. Hypothermia in the treatment of large MCA strokes

Hypothermia has also been evaluated in the treatment of cerebral edema after large MCA infarctions. Schwab and collaborators induced moderate hypothermia in 25 patients with large MCA strokes.[58] Hypothermia was induced within 14 ± 7 hours after stroke onset by external cooling with cooling blankets, cold infusions, and cold washing. Hypothermia at 33°C body-core temperature was maintained for 48 to 72 hours, and intracranial pressure (ICP), cerebral perfusion pressure, and brain temperature were continuously monitored. Elevated ICP values were significantly reduced during hypothermia. Herniation caused by a secondary rise in ICP after rewarming was the cause of death in most patients. The most frequent complication of moderate hypothermia was pneumonia in 10 of the 25 patients [40%). Authors concluded that moderate hypothermia can help to control critically elevated ICP values in severe space-occupying edema after MCA stroke. This and a similar study by the same group were pivotal in demonstrating that hypothermia was safe and effective in the treatment of increased ICP after malignant MCA infarction.[59]

A prospective study performed by the same group, induced hypothermia in 50 patients with cooling blankets as well as alcohol and ice bags within 22 ± 9 hours after stroke onset.[59] Hypothermia was maintained for 24 to 72 hours and passive rewarming performed over a mean duration of 17 hours. Time required for cooling to < 33°C varied from 3.5 to 11 hours. The most frequent complications of hypothermic therapy were thrombocytopenia (70%). Faster rewarming (< 16 hours) was associated with rebound increased ICP, and most deaths occurred during the rewarming period. Further data in MCA infarct patients suggests that controlled rewarming rates of ≤ 0.1 per hour allow for improved control of ICP when compared with patients in whom rewarming is achieved in an uncontrolled fashion.[60]

Georgiadis and collaborators compared hypothermia with hemicraniectomy in the treatment of more than 2/3 of the MCA infarction.[61] Seventeen patients underwent hemicraniectomy and 19 were treated with moderate hypothermia (33°C), which was induced with cooling blankets and endovascular devices. Hypothermia was induced for 71 ± 21 hours (range, 24 - 116 hours), whereas duration of rewarming varied between 25 and 34 hours. Prolongation of hypothermia >72 hours was always related to raised ICP during rewarming attempts. Mortality was 12% in the hemicraniectomy group and 47% in the hypothermia group; one patient treated with hypothermia died as a result of cooling complications (sepsis) and three patients died of ICP crises that occurred during rewarming.

Another small prospective study with 25 patients compared hypothermia with hemicraniectomy and hemicraniectomy alone in the treatment of patients with large MCA strokes.[62] Hemicraniectomy was performed within 15 +/- 6 h after the ischemic event, followed by hypothermia. There were no severe side effects of hypothermia. Patients treated with hemicraniectomy plus moderate hypothermia had a tendency to better outcome after 6 months when compared to patients treated with hemicraniectomy alone.

9. Human studies of hypothermia in hemorrhagic stroke

ICH accounts for approximately 10% of strokes and the 30-day mortality rate is approximately 52%.[63] After the acute phase of ICH, high morbidity and mortality are essentially caused by the evolution of a peri-hemorrhagic, space-occupying edema associated with gradually increasing ICP.[64] Although the natural course of edema formation is still not fully understood, edema mostly increases during the first week and reaches its maximum during the second week after bleeding onset.[65, 66] Animal studies have suggested that hypothermia may have a neuroprotective role after ICH in reducing edema formation by various mechanisms.[67, 68]

One of the first experiences with hypothermia in the treatment of ICH was reported by Howell and collaborators in 1956.[69] Hypothermia between 30°C to 32°C was induced in eight patients with spontaneous ICH. Although signs of herniation improved in all patients, six patients died from systemic complications, most commonly aspiration. Anecdotally, hypothermia was induced with ice bags, alcohol, and even opening the windows in the middle of the Canadian winter.

Kollmar and collaborators treated twelve patients with supratentorial large ICH (> 25 mL) with hypothermia (35°C) for 10 days.[5] In the hypothermia group, edema volume remained stable during 14 days, whereas edema significantly increased in the control group. However, pneumonia was more frequent in the hypothermia group. Based on these results, the same investigators planned the Cooling in Intracerebral Hemorrhage (CINCH) trial. [70] This is a prospective multicenter trial that WILL enroll 50 patients with large ICH and randomly assign them to mild hypothermia versus conventional medical management.

Ischemic Stroke

Authors	Study	Number of Patients	Time from Stroke	Cooling Technique	Cooling Time	Patient	Anti-shivering	Target Temp	Time to Target Temp	Complications	Comment
Kammersgaard (43) (2000)	Single center, nonrandomized, open label.	17	12 h	Surface	6 h	Non-intubated	Meperidine	35.5°C	6 h	Infection 18%	Awake patients tolerated surface hypothermia.
Keller (44) (2000)	Single center, nonrandomized, open label.	6	63.5 h	Surface	48-96 h	Intubated	Midazolam, fentanyl and atracurium.	33°C	NA	NA	Hypothermia decreased $CMRO_2$ and CBF.
Georgiadis (45) (2001)	Single center, nonrandomized, open label.	6	28±17 h	Endovascular	48-72 h	Intubated	Midazolam, fentanyl and atracurium.	33°C	3±1 h	Bradycardia 50% Pneumonia 100% Hypotension 100% Thromb 33%	Induction and maintenance of hypothermia with intravenous cooling was feasible.
Krieger (46) (2001)	Single center, nonrandomized, open label, parallel control (COOL AID)	10	6 h	Surface	12-72 h	Intubated	Propofol and atracurium.	33°C	3.5± 1.5 h	Bradycardia 50% Arrythmia 30% Hypotension 30%	Hypothermia was well tolerated after thrombolysis.
De Georgia (47) (2004)	Multicenter, randomized, open label. (COOL AID)	18	12 h	Endovascular	24 h	Non-intubated	Air warming blanket, buspirone and meperidine.	33°C	77± 44 min	Pneumonia 11% Arrythmia 11% Retroperitoneal hematoma 5%	Endovascular hypothermia in awake patients was well tolerated.
Lyden (48) (2005)	Multicenter, open label, nonrandomized. (ICTuS)	18	12 h	Endovascular	12-24 h	Non-intubated	Air warming blanket, buspirone and meperidine.	33°C	7 h	DVT 22% Bradycardia 22% Hypokalemia 22% Groin hematoma 11% Arrythmia 11%	Endovascular hypothermia in awake patients was well tolerated.
Martin-Schild (52) (2009)	Single center, nonrandomized, open label.	18	5 h	Surface and endovascular	24 h	Non-intubated	Air warming blanket, buspirone and meperidine.	33-35°C	8 h	Pneumonia 20%	Hypothermia was combined with caffeinol and tPA in nonintubated patients.
Hemmen (50) (2010)	Multicenter, randomized, double-blinded. (ICTuS-L)	28	6 h	Endovascular	24 h	Non-intubated	Air warming blanket, buspirone and meperidine.	33°C	7 h	Pneumonia 25% DVT 14%	Hypothermia was well tolerated after thrombolysis. 24-h assessments were affected by sedation in the hypothermia group.

	Authors	Study	Number of Patients	Time from Stroke	Cooling Technique	Cooling Time	Patient	Anti-shivering	Target Temp	Time to Target Temp	Complications	Comment
MCA Stroke	Schwab (58) (1998)	Single center, nonrandomized, open label.	25	14±7 h	Surface	48-72 h	Intubated	Fentanyl, propofol and atracurium.	33°C	14±4 h	Pneumonia 10% Arrythmia 60%	Hypothermia effective in the treatment of increased ICP after MCA infarction.
	Schwab (59) (1998)	Single center, nonrandomized, open label.	50	22±9 h	Surface	48-72 h	Intubated	Fentanyl, midazolam or propofol and atracurium.	33°C	22 ± 3.5 - 11 h	Thromb 70% Bradycardia 62% Pneumonia 48%	Fast rewarming was associated with rebound increased ICP.
	Georgiadis (61) (2002)	Single center, nonrandomized, open label.	19	24 h	Surface and endovascular	48-72 h	Intubated	Fentanyl, midazolam and atracurium.	33°C	4 ± 1 h	Pneumonia 78% Arrythmia 42% Bradycardia 58% Thromb 37% Hypokalemia 26%	Hypothermia was compared with hemicraniectomy in the treatment of large MCA strokes. The hypothermia group had higher mortality due to increased ICP during rewarming.
	Els (62) (2006)	Single center, randomized, open label.	12	NA	Surface and endovascular	48 h	Intubated	Fentanyl and midazolam.	35°C	2 ± 1 h	Bradycardia 8%	Hypothermia was used with hemicraniectomy.
Hemorrhagic Stroke	Kollmar (70) (2010)	Single center, nonrandomized, open label.	12	12 h	Endovascular	10 d	Intubated	Sufentanyl, midazolam, meperidine and cisatracurium	35°C	NA	Pneumonia 100% Thromb 33% Bradycardia 25%	Hypothermia decreased perihematomal edema.

Temp = temperature; thromb = thrombocytopenia; $CMRO_2$ = Cerebral metabolic rate of oxigen; CBF = cerebral blood flow; tPA = tissue plasminogen activator; ICP = intracranial pressure; MCA = middle cerebral artery; NA = not available; h = hour, d = day; min = minutes.

Table 1. Main studies of the use of hypothermia in the treatment of acute stroke.

Hypothermia has also been evaluated in the management of subarachnoid hemorrhage (SAH). Gasser and collaborators treated 21 patients with poor grade SAH and cerebral edema with long-term hypothermia (>72 hrs).[71] Nine patients were treated for <72 hrs and 12 for >72 hrs. Functional independence at 3 months was achieved in 48% of patients, but the outcome did not differ with the group of patients treated without hypothermia. The most common form of complication was infection in both groups.

10. Complications of hypothermia

Induced therapeutic hypothermia is an intensive care procedure that has to be performed under continuous monitoring. Since most patients who are cooled are critically ill, they may be more prone to develop complications. These complications appear to be associated with de degree of hypothermia, with the risk of side effects being correlated with prolonged hypothermia and lower temperatures. In general, hypothermia is well tolerated, but complications may include: 1) cardiac: arrhythmias, bradycardia, reduced ventricular contractility, and hypotension; 2) immunologic: immunosuppression; 3) hematologic: thrombocytopenia and mild coagulopathy; and 4) metabolic: shivering, hyperglycemia, hypokalemia, ileus, and cold-induced diuresis. The most common complication in reported studies is pneumonia, followed by asymptomatic bradycardia, cardiac arrhythmias and thrombocytopenia (table).[14]

Pneumonia appears to occur more frequently in intubated patients who undergo cooling. Endovascular cooling with use of warm blankets to reduce shivering and prevent intubation is an alternative to surface cooling and may reduce the rate of pneumonia.

The most dangerous phase of induced hypothermia is the rewarming period. Particular care is required in stroke patients with intracranial mass effect and elevated ICP. Overly rapid rewarming can lead to a systemic inflammatory response syndrome; with systemic vasodilatation, hypotension, and reflex ICP elevation.[14] As a general rule, hypothermia patients with increased ICP should undergo active controlled rewarming (or "decooling") at a rate of 0.1°C per hour. Faster rates of 0.25°C to 0.33°C per hour can be tolerated in patients without ICP issues.[72-74] This high ICP rebound has especially been observed in patients with malignant MCA infarctions.[75]

One common complication of hypothermia that usually is overlooked is sedation. It has been demonstrated that patients who undergo hypothermia are more likely to receive sedation than those who are not treated with hypothermia.[76] Sedation in hypothermia patients may linger longer in the system, confounding neurological examination and prognostication.[77] This becomes a relevant issue in stroke patients who require daily neurological assessments.

11. Conclusion and recommendations

Despite the many potential neuroprotective effects of hypothermia seen in animal stroke models and the benefit of hypothermia observed in humans following cardiac arrest, there is still no solid evidence demonstrating improved outcomes in stroke patients. In addition, a systematic review found no definitive evidence that either physical or chemical cooling interventions improve outcomes after acute ischemic stroke.[78] The total number of participants included in the studies reviewed in this chapter is far to small and the interventions too heterogeneous for definitive conclusions (table). Moreover, all studies were designed to test safety and feasibility, and allowed rather long time periods between stroke onset and start of cooling, which may lower the likelihood of observing a treatment effect.

Stroke studies have used surface and endovascular cooling systems for induction and maintenance of hypothermia (table). Goal temperatures usually range from 33° to 35°C. IV infusion of ice-cold saline [25 mL/kg body weight) has been shown to induce hypothermia rapidly and may be used as an initial cooling method in stroke patients who are initially assessed in the field.[53]

Pharmacologic agents like meperidine and buspirone, and concurrent skin warming inhibit shivering and allow patients to tolerate treatment with less sedation. Moreover, these anti-shivering protocols have allowed the induction and maintenance of mild and moderate hypothermia in awake patients.[47] Recent studies have demonstrated that endovascular cooling is more accurate in keeping patients in the target temperature range than surface cooling with ice bags and cooling blankets.[79, 80] Endovascular cooling also allows for concurrent use of surface warming to reduce shivering. However, endovascular cooling implies accessing the femoral vein to place the cooling catheter, increasing the risk of procedural complications and infection. In general, each center should choose the cooling method that is more familiar to the personnel and easier to implement.

Similar uncertainty exists on the optimal treatment duration. In animal models of focal cerebral ischemia, pathophysiological processes exert their deleterious effects over various time courses, extending from the first hours to several days after vessel occlusion.[81] Such observations may imply that temperature lowering therapy should be more effective when used for prolonged time. On the other hand, longer treatment was not associated with improved outcomes in a meta-analysis of hypothermia in animal models of focal cerebral ischemia. Moreover, the risk of side effects such as infections may increase with longer cooling times.[39] In clinical trials of cardiac arrest, hypothermia was maintained for 12 or 24 hours.[3] Most recent studies of hypothermia in acute ischemic stroke aim for 12 – 24 hours of cooling (table).

For unknown reasons, patients with massive brain injuries may experience rebound intracranial hypertension when rapidly rewarmed after prolonged periods of mild to moderate hypothermia. Whether this occurs in experimental stroke models has not been widely studied. Previous stroke studies suggest that controlled rewarming seems to prevent rebound brain edema and is the standard protocol in most recent trials.[14] Trials using milder hypothermia [35°C) and slower rewarming periods have reported lower complication rates.[62] For practical purposes, a 24-hour cooling period followed by a >12-hour slow rewarming, such as 0.1° C/h is advised.[82]

Author details

Edgar A. Samaniego
Baptist Neuroscience Center, Baptist Cardiac and Vascular Institute, Miami, Florida, USA

12. References

[1] Adams HP, Jr., Bendixen BH, Kappelle LJ, Biller J, Love BB, Gordon DL, et al. Classification of subtype of acute ischemic stroke. Definitions for use in a multicenter clinical trial. TOAST. Trial of Org 10172 in Acute Stroke Treatment. Stroke. 1993 Jan;24(1):35-41.

[2] O'Collins VE, Macleod MR, Donnan GA, Horky LL, van der Worp BH, Howells DW. 1,026 experimental treatments in acute stroke. Ann Neurol. 2006 Mar;59(3):467-77.

[3] Bernard SA, Gray TW, Buist MD, Jones BM, Silvester W, Gutteridge G, et al. Treatment of comatose survivors of out-of-hospital cardiac arrest with induced hypothermia. N Engl J Med. 2002 Feb 21;346(8):557-63.

[4] Gluckman PD, Wyatt JS, Azzopardi D, Ballard R, Edwards AD, Ferriero DM, et al. Selective head cooling with mild systemic hypothermia after neonatal encephalopathy: multicentre randomised trial. Lancet. 2005 Feb 19-25;365(9460):663-70.

[5] Kollmar R, Staykov D, D√∂rfler A, Schellinger PD, Schwab S, Bardutzky Jr. Hypothermia Reduces Perihemorrhagic Edema After Intracerebral Hemorrhage. Stroke. [10.1161/STROKEAHA.110.587758]. 2010;41(8):1684-9.

[6] Hammer MD, Krieger DW. Hypothermia for acute ischemic stroke: not just another neuroprotectant. Neurologist. 2003 Nov;9(6):280-9.

[7] Lee JM, Grabb MC, Zipfel GJ, Choi DW. Brain tissue responses to ischemia. J Clin Invest. 2000 Sep;106(6):723-31.

[8] Nishijima MK, Koehler RC, Hurn PD, Eleff SM, Norris S, Jacobus WE, et al. Postischemic recovery rate of cerebral ATP, phosphocreatine, pH, and evoked potentials. Am J Physiol. 1989 Dec;257(6 Pt 2):H1860-70.

[9] Kintner D, Costello DJ, Levin AB, Gilboe DD. Brain metabolism after 30 minutes of hypoxic or anoxic perfusion or ischemia. Am J Physiol. 1980 Dec;239(6):E501-9.

[10] Busch E, Kruger K, Allegrini PR, Kerskens CM, Gyngell ML, Hoehn-Berlage M, et al. Reperfusion after thrombolytic therapy of embolic stroke in the rat: magnetic resonance and biochemical imaging. J Cereb Blood Flow Metab. 1998 Apr;18(4):407-18.

[11] Yenari MA, Colbourne F, Hemmen TM, Han HS, Krieger D. Therapeutic hypothermia in stroke. Stroke Res Treat. 2011;2011:157969.

[12] Berger C, Schabitz WR, Georgiadis D, Steiner T, Aschoff A, Schwab S. Effects of hypothermia on excitatory amino acids and metabolism in stroke patients: a microdialysis study. Stroke. 2002 Feb;33(2):519-24.

[13] Globus MY, Alonso O, Dietrich WD, Busto R, Ginsberg MD. Glutamate release and free radical production following brain injury: effects of posttraumatic hypothermia. J Neurochem. 1995 Oct;65(4):1704-11.

[14] Linares G, Mayer SA. Hypothermia for the treatment of ischemic and hemorrhagic stroke. Crit Care Med. 2009 Jul;37(7 Suppl):S243-9.

[15] Ji X, Luo Y, Ling F, Stetler RA, Lan J, Cao G, et al. Mild hypothermia diminishes oxidative DNA damage and pro-death signaling events after cerebral ischemia: a mechanism for neuroprotection. Front Biosci. 2007;12:1737-47.

[16] Feigin VL, Anderson CS, Rodgers A, Anderson NE, Gunn AJ. The emerging role of induced hypothermia in the management of acute stroke. J Clin Neurosci. 2002 Sep;9(5):502-7.

[17] Steen PA, Newberg L, Milde JH, Michenfelder JD. Hypothermia and barbiturates: individual and combined effects on canine cerebral oxygen consumption. Anesthesiology. 1983 Jun;58(6):527-32.

[18] Liu L, Yenari MA. Therapeutic hypothermia: neuroprotective mechanisms. Front Biosci. 2007;12:816-25.

[19] Yenari M, Kitagawa K, Lyden P, Perez-Pinzon M. Metabolic downregulation: a key to successful neuroprotection? Stroke. 2008 Oct;39(10):2910-7.

[20] Wagner S, Nagel S, Kluge B, Schwab S, Heiland S, Koziol J, et al. Topographically graded postischemic presence of metalloproteinases is inhibited by hypothermia. Brain Res. 2003 Sep 12;984(1-2):63-75.

[21] Hamann GF, Burggraf D, Martens HK, Liebetrau M, Jager G, Wunderlich N, et al. Mild to moderate hypothermia prevents microvascular basal lamina antigen loss in experimental focal cerebral ischemia. Stroke. 2004 Mar;35(3):764-9.

[22] Lee JE, Yoon YJ, Moseley ME, Yenari MA. Reduction in levels of matrix metalloproteinases and increased expression of tissue inhibitor of metalloproteinase-2 in response to mild hypothermia therapy in experimental stroke. J Neurosurg. 2005 Aug;103(2):289-97.

[23] Horstmann S, Koziol JA, Martinez-Torres F, Nagel S, Gardner H, Wagner S. Sonographic monitoring of mass effect in stroke patients treated with hypothermia. Correlation with intracranial pressure and matrix metalloproteinase 2 and 9 expression. J Neurol Sci. 2009 Jan 15;276(1-2):75-8.

[24] Ohta H, Terao Y, Shintani Y, Kiyota Y. Therapeutic time window of post-ischemic mild hypothermia and the gene expression associated with the neuroprotection in rat focal cerebral ischemia. Neurosci Res. 2007 Mar;57(3):424-33.

[25] Han HS, Qiao Y, Karabiyikoglu M, Giffard RG, Yenari MA. Influence of mild hypothermia on inducible nitric oxide synthase expression and reactive nitrogen production in experimental stroke and inflammation. J Neurosci. 2002 May 15;22(10):3921-8.

[26] Xu L, Yenari MA, Steinberg GK, Giffard RG. Mild hypothermia reduces apoptosis of mouse neurons in vitro early in the cascade. J Cereb Blood Flow Metab. 2002 Jan;22(1):21-8.

[27] Van Hemelrijck A, Hachimi-Idrissi S, Sarre S, Ebinger G, Michotte Y. Post-ischaemic mild hypothermia inhibits apoptosis in the penumbral region by reducing neuronal nitric oxide synthase activity and thereby preventing endothelin-1-induced hydroxyl radical formation. Eur J Neurosci. 2005 Sep;22(6):1327-37.

[28] Zhao H, Shimohata T, Wang JQ, Sun G, Schaal DW, Sapolsky RM, et al. Akt contributes to neuroprotection by hypothermia against cerebral ischemia in rats. J Neurosci. 2005 Oct 19;25(42):9794-806.
[29] D'Cruz BJ, Fertig KC, Filiano AJ, Hicks SD, DeFranco DB, Callaway CW. Hypothermic reperfusion after cardiac arrest augments brain-derived neurotrophic factor activation. J Cereb Blood Flow Metab. 2002 Jul;22(7):843-51.
[30] Schmidt KM, Repine MJ, Hicks SD, DeFranco DB, Callaway CW. Regional changes in glial cell line-derived neurotrophic factor after cardiac arrest and hypothermia in rats. Neurosci Lett. 2004 Sep 23;368(2):135-9.
[31] Boris-Moller F, Kamme F, Wieloch T. The effect of hypothermia on the expression of neurotrophin mRNA in the hippocampus following transient cerebral ischemia in the rat. Brain Res Mol Brain Res. 1998 Dec 10;63(1):163-73.
[32] Vosler PS, Logue ES, Repine MJ, Callaway CW. Delayed hypothermia preferentially increases expression of brain-derived neurotrophic factor exon III in rat hippocampus after asphyxial cardiac arrest. Brain Res Mol Brain Res. 2005 Apr 27;135(1-2):21-9.
[33] Zhao H, Yenari MA, Cheng D, Sapolsky RM, Steinberg GK. Biphasic cytochrome c release after transient global ischemia and its inhibition by hypothermia. J Cereb Blood Flow Metab. 2005 Sep;25(9):1119-29.
[34] Zhang Z, Sobel RA, Cheng D, Steinberg GK, Yenari MA. Mild hypothermia increases Bcl-2 protein expression following global cerebral ischemia. Brain Res Mol Brain Res. 2001 Nov 1;95(1-2):75-85.
[35] Yenari MA, Iwayama S, Cheng D, Sun GH, Fujimura M, Morita-Fujimura Y, et al. Mild hypothermia attenuates cytochrome c release but does not alter Bcl-2 expression or caspase activation after experimental stroke. J Cereb Blood Flow Metab. 2002 Jan;22(1):29-38.
[36] Inamasu J, Suga S, Sato S, Horiguchi T, Akaji K, Mayanagi K, et al. Postischemic hypothermia attenuates apoptotic cell death in transient focal ischemia in rats. Acta Neurochir Suppl. 2000;76:525-7.
[37] Prakasa Babu P, Yoshida Y, Su M, Segura M, Kawamura S, Yasui N. Immunohistochemical expression of Bcl-2, Bax and cytochrome c following focal cerebral ischemia and effect of hypothermia in rat. Neurosci Lett. 2000 Sep 22;291(3):196-200.
[38] Polderman KH, Herold I. Therapeutic hypothermia and controlled normothermia in the intensive care unit: practical considerations, side effects, and cooling methods. Crit Care Med. 2009 Mar;37(3):1101-20.
[39] van der Worp HB, Sena ES, Donnan GA, Howells DW, Macleod MR. Hypothermia in animal models of acute ischaemic stroke: a systematic review and meta-analysis. Brain. 2007 Dec;130(Pt 12):3063-74.
[40] Boysen G, Christensen H. Stroke severity determines body temperature in acute stroke. Stroke. 2001 Feb;32(2):413-7.
[41] Chopp M, Welch KM, Tidwell CD, Knight R, Helpern JA. Effect of mild hyperthermia on recovery of metabolic function after global cerebral ischemia in cats. Stroke. 1988 Dec;19(12):1521-5.

[42] Reith J, Jorgensen HS, Pedersen PM, Nakayama H, Raaschou HO, Jeppesen LL, et al. Body temperature in acute stroke: relation to stroke severity, infarct size, mortality, and outcome. Lancet. 1996 Feb 17;347(8999):422-5.
[43] Kammersgaard LP, Rasmussen BH, Jorgensen HS, Reith J, Weber U, Olsen TS. Feasibility and safety of inducing modest hypothermia in awake patients with acute stroke through surface cooling: A case-control study: the Copenhagen Stroke Study. Stroke. 2000 Sep;31(9):2251-6.
[44] Keller E, Steiner T, Fandino J, Schwab S, Hacke W. Changes in cerebral blood flow and oxygen metabolism during moderate hypothermia in patients with severe middle cerebral artery infarction. Neurosurg Focus. 2000;8(5):e4.
[45] Georgiadis D, Schwarz S, Kollmar R, Schwab S. Endovascular cooling for moderate hypothermia in patients with acute stroke: first results of a novel approach. Stroke. 2001 Nov;32(11):2550-3.
[46] Krieger DW, De Georgia MA, Abou-Chebl A, Andrefsky JC, Sila CA, Katzan IL, et al. Cooling for acute ischemic brain damage (cool aid): an open pilot study of induced hypothermia in acute ischemic stroke. Stroke. 2001 Aug;32(8):1847-54.
[47] De Georgia MA, Krieger DW, Abou-Chebl A, Devlin TG, Jauss M, Davis SM, et al. Cooling for Acute Ischemic Brain Damage (COOL AID): a feasibility trial of endovascular cooling. Neurology. 2004 Jul 27;63(2):312-7.
[48] Lyden PD, Allgren RL, Ng K, Akins P, Meyer B, Al-Sanani F, et al. Intravascular Cooling in the Treatment of Stroke (ICTuS): early clinical experience. J Stroke Cerebrovasc Dis. 2005 May-Jun;14(3):107-14.
[49] Guluma KZ, Oh H, Yu SW, Meyer BC, Rapp K, Lyden PD. Effect of endovascular hypothermia on acute ischemic edema: morphometric analysis of the ICTuS trial. Neurocrit Care. 2008;8(1):42-7.
[50] Hemmen TM, Raman R, Guluma KZ, Meyer BC, Gomes JA, Cruz-Flores S, et al. Intravenous thrombolysis plus hypothermia for acute treatment of ischemic stroke (ICTuS-L): final results. Stroke. 2010 Oct;41(10):2265-70.
[51] Hemmen TM, Lyden PD. Induced Hypothermia for Acute Stroke. Stroke. [10.1161/01.STR.0000247920.15708.fa]. 2007;38(2):794-9.
[52] Martin-Schild S, Hallevi H, Shaltoni H, Barreto AD, Gonzales NR, Aronowski J, et al. Combined neuroprotective modalities coupled with thrombolysis in acute ischemic stroke: a pilot study of caffeinol and mild hypothermia. Journal of Stroke and Cerebrovascular Diseases: The Official Journal of National Stroke Association. [10.1016/j.jstrokecerebrovasdis.2008.09.015]. 2009;18(2):86-96.
[53] Kollmar R, Schellinger PD, Steigleder T, Kohrmann M, Schwab S. Ice-cold saline for the induction of mild hypothermia in patients with acute ischemic stroke: a pilot study. Stroke. 2009 May;40(5):1907-9.
[54] Hemmen TM, Lyden PD. Induced hypothermia for acute stroke. Stroke. 2007 Feb;38(2 Suppl):794-9.
[55] Yenari MA, Palmer JT, Bracci PM, Steinberg GK. Thrombolysis with tissue plasminogen activator (tPA) is temperature dependent. Thromb Res. 1995 Mar 1;77(5):475-81.

[56] Naess H, Idicula T, Lagallo N, Brogger J, Waje-Andreassen U, Thomassen L. Inverse relationship of baseline body temperature and outcome between ischemic stroke patients treated and not treated with thrombolysis: the Bergen stroke study. Acta Neurol Scand. 2010 Dec;122(6):414-7.
[57] Lees JS, Mishra NK, Saini M, Lyden PD, Shuaib A. Low body temperature does not compromise the treatment effect of alteplase. Stroke. 2011 Sep;42(9):2618-21.
[58] Schwab S, Schwarz S, Spranger M, Keller E, Bertram M, Hacke W. Moderate hypothermia in the treatment of patients with severe middle cerebral artery infarction. Stroke. 1998 Dec;29(12):2461-6.
[59] Schwab S, Georgiadis D, Berrouschot Jr, Schellinger PD, Graffagnino C, Mayer SA. Feasibility and Safety of Moderate Hypothermia After Massive Hemispheric Infarction. Stroke. [10.1161/hs0901.095394]. 2001;32(9):2033-5.
[60] Steiner T, Friede T, Aschoff A, Schellinger PD, Schwab S, Hacke W. Effect and feasibility of controlled rewarming after moderate hypothermia in stroke patients with malignant infarction of the middle cerebral artery. Stroke; a Journal of Cerebral Circulation. 2001;32(12):2833-5.
[61] Georgiadis D, Schwarz S, Aschoff A, Schwab S. Hemicraniectomy and moderate hypothermia in patients with severe ischemic stroke. Stroke. 2002 Jun;33(6):1584-8.
[62] Els T, Oehm E, Voigt S, Klisch J, Hetzel A, Kassubek J. Safety and therapeutical benefit of hemicraniectomy combined with mild hypothermia in comparison with hemicraniectomy alone in patients with malignant ischemic stroke. Cerebrovasc Dis. 2006;21(1-2):79-85.
[63] Broderick J, Connolly S, Feldmann E, Hanley D, Kase C, Krieger D, et al. Guidelines for the management of spontaneous intracerebral hemorrhage in adults: 2007 update: a guideline from the American Heart Association/American Stroke Association Stroke Council, High Blood Pressure Research Council, and the Quality of Care and Outcomes in Research Interdisciplinary Working Group. Circulation. [10.1161/CIRCULATIONAHA.107.183689]. 2007;116(16):e391-413-e391-413.
[64] Zazulia AR, Diringer MN, Derdeyn CP, Powers WJ. Progression of mass effect after intracerebral hemorrhage. Stroke; a Journal of Cerebral Circulation. 1999;30(6):1167-73.
[65] Inaji M, Tomita H, Tone O, Tamaki M, Suzuki R, Ohno K. Chronological changes of perihematomal edema of human intracerebral hematoma. Acta Neurochirurgica Supplement. 2003;86:445-8.
[66] Venkatasubramanian C, Mlynash M, Finley-Caulfield A, Eyngorn I, Kalimuthu R, Snider RW, et al. Natural History of Perihematomal Edema After Intracerebral Hemorrhage Measured by Serial Magnetic Resonance Imaging. Stroke. [10.1161/STROKEAHA.110.590646]. 2011;42(1):73-80.
[67] MacLellan CL, Davies LM, Fingas MS, Colbourne F. The influence of hypothermia on outcome after intracerebral hemorrhage in rats. Stroke; a Journal of Cerebral Circulation. [10.1161/01.STR.0000217268.81963.78]. 2006;37(5):1266-70.
[68] Kawanishi M, Kawai N, Nakamura T, Luo C, Tamiya T, Nagao S. Effect of delayed mild brain hypothermia on edema formation after intracerebral hemorrhage in rats. Journal

of Stroke and Cerebrovascular Diseases: The Official Journal of National Stroke Association. [10.1016/j.jstrokecerebrovasdis.2008.01.003]. 2008;17(4):187-95.
[69] Howell DA, Posnikoff J, Stratford JG. Prolonged hypothermia in treatment of massive cerebral haemorrhage; a preliminary report. Canadian Medical Association Journal. 1956;75(5):388-94.
[70] Kollmar R, Juettler E, Huttner HB, D√∂rfler A, Staykov D, Kallmuenzer B, et al. Cooling in intracerebral hemorrhage (CINCH) trial: protocol of a randomized German-Austrian clinical trial. International Journal of Stroke: Official Journal of the International Stroke Society. [10.1111/j.1747-4949.2011.00707.x]. 2012;7(2):168-72.
[71] Gasser S, Khan N, Yonekawa Y, Imhof HG, Keller E. Long-term hypothermia in patients with severe brain edema after poor-grade subarachnoid hemorrhage: feasibility and intensive care complications. J Neurosurg Anesthesiol. 2003 Jul;15(3):240-8.
[72] Krieger DW, Georgia D, A M, Abou-Chebl A, Andrefsky JC, Sila CA, et al. Cooling for Acute Ischemic Brain Damage (COOL AID) An Open Pilot Study of Induced Hypothermia in Acute Ischemic Stroke. Stroke. [10.1161/01.STR.32.8.1847]. 2001;32(8):1847-54.
[73] Ginsberg MD, Sternau LL, Globus MY, Dietrich WD, Busto R. Therapeutic modulation of brain temperature: relevance to ischemic brain injury. Cerebrovascular and Brain Metabolism Reviews. 1992;4(3):189-225.
[74] Krieger DW, Yenari MA. Therapeutic hypothermia for acute ischemic stroke: what do laboratory studies teach us? Stroke. 2004 Jun;35(6):1482-9.
[75] Steiner T, Friede T, Aschoff A, Schellinger PD, Schwab S, Hacke W. Effect and feasibility of controlled rewarming after moderate hypothermia in stroke patients with malignant infarction of the middle cerebral artery. Stroke. 2001 Dec 1;32(12):2833-5.
[76] Samaniego EA, Mlynash M, Caulfield AF, Eyngorn I, Wijman CAC. Sedation confounds outcome prediction in cardiac arrest survivors treated with hypothermia. Neurocritical Care. [10.1007/s12028-010-9412-8]. 2011;15(1):113-9.
[77] Samaniego EA, Persoon S, Wijman CAC. Prognosis after cardiac arrest and hypothermia: a new paradigm. Current Neurology and Neuroscience Reports. [10.1007/s11910-010-0148-9]. 2011;11(1):111-9.
[78] Den Hertog HM, van der Worp HB, Tseng MC, Dippel DW. Cooling therapy for acute stroke. Cochrane Database Syst Rev. 2009(1):CD001247.
[79] Gillies MA, Pratt R, Whiteley C, Borg J, Beale RJ, Tibby SM. Therapeutic hypothermia after cardiac arrest: a retrospective comparison of surface and endovascular cooling techniques. Resuscitation. [10.1016/j.resuscitation.2010.05.001]. 2010;81(9):1117-22.
[80] Finley Caulfield A, Rachabattula S, Eyngorn I, Hamilton SA, Kalimuthu R, Hsia AW, et al. A Comparison of Cooling Techniques to Treat Cardiac Arrest Patients with Hypothermia. Stroke Research and Treatment. [10.4061/2011/690506]. 2011;2011:1-6.
[81] Dirnagl U, Iadecola C, Moskowitz MA. Pathobiology of ischaemic stroke: an integrated view. Trends Neurosci. 1999 Sep;22(9):391-7.
[82] Krieger DW, Yenari MA. Therapeutic hypothermia for acute ischemic stroke: what do laboratory studies teach us? Stroke; a Journal of Cerebral Circulation. [10.1161/01.STR.0000126118.44249.5c]. 2004;35(6):1482-9.

Chapter 5

Hypothermia for Intracerebral Hemorrhage, Subarachnoid Hemorrhage & Spinal Cord Injury

David E. Tannehill

Additional information is available at the end of the chapter

http://dx.doi.org/10.5772/54925

1. Introduction

As described previously in this book, hypothermia likely has many positive effects on injured brain and spinal cord to limit the damage caused by secondary injury. This secondary injury has multiple mechanisms, including inflammation, excitotoxicity, calcium homeostasis, blood brain barrier damage, release of toxic intermediates including free radicals, as well as cell necrosis & apoptosis (1). Hypothermia has been shown to be an effective treatment for comatose survivors of out of hospital cardiac arrest to both improve mortality and neurologic outcomes (2, 3). Much less is known about the role of hypothermia for treating patients that have suffered an intracerebral or subarachnoid hemorrhage. Experience and literature on the subject is quite limited. The same is true for hypothermia in the treatment of acute spinal cord injury. In fact, data on this topic is even more limited.

However, in the coming years it is likely that we will see more research on this important topic. The technology available to clinicians for achieving the treatment goals of this strategy has rapidly expanded in the past decade. Additionally, its ease of use and increasing familiarity amongst clinicians and intensive care unit staff will only help in growing the field. The basic science background, while not extensive, is at least encouraging and it is expanding. The clinical use, or at least consideration of this therapy is slowly beginning to expand as well. Options for medical therapy to improve outcomes in ICH, SAH & SCI are limited. Hopefully this continued work will improve upon that. This chapter will explore what has been published on these topics to this point.

2. Therapeutic hypothermia for acute spinal cord injury

In the 1960's and 1970's, multiple investigators published data examining the possibility of employing hypothermic therapy to improve outcomes in acute spinal cord injury. At that time, most of the studies focused on local cooling via the administration of cold saline to the spinal cord during decompressive laminectomy and durotomy (4-6). However, these studies were not rigorous randomized controlled trials and were fraught with multiple confounders, such as the concomitant administration of corticosteroids and the potential effects of surgery itself (7,8). This, combined with the technical difficulty and invasive nature of local cooling, lead to the general abandonment of the idea.

As technology improved and our understanding of the possible beneficial effects of systemic hypothermia grew, so did interest in applying this strategy to the acute spinal cord injury patient (9,10). Multiple animal studies have suggested a positive effect of either locally or systemically applied therapeutic hypothermia (9). However, clinical experience in the modern era is minimal. In 2010, there was a high-profile case of an NFL football player suspected to have a spinal cord injury who was treated with systemic hypothermia (11). This case garnered the attention of the mass media in addition to the medical community. However, it is important to recognize that it is impossible to discern if this patient's excellent outcome can be in any way attributed to therapeutic hypothermia. That case does add to the literature describing the safe use of targeted temperature therapy in acute spinal cord injury. The largest and most often quoted case series for therapeutic hypothermia in this patient population is a retrospective review described by Levi et al in 2009 (12). This group describes their institutional experience with therapeutic hypothermia in 14 adult patients with acute, complete cervical spinal cord injury who presented to their institution over a two year period. Only complete cervical spinal cord injury patients with a GCS 15 were considered for their hypothermia treatment protocol. An intravascular cooling device was used to achieve and maintain a core body temperature of 33°C over a 48 hour period. Corticosteroids were not used. All patients underwent surgical intervention. Patients were then rewarmed over a 24-32hr period. This group of patients averaged 39.4 years old from a range of 16-62years. Induction of hypothermia began within 9.17+/-2.24hr and time to target temperature was 2.72+/-0.42hr. They documented a strong correlation between temperature and heart rate. Additionally, in one patient, CSF temperature was measured and found to closely approximate core temperature. Importantly, none of the 14 patients suffered a life-threatening adverse event attributable to therapeutic hypothermia. The adverse events described were primarily respiratory and closely approximated the type and rate of adverse events experienced in an historical control cohort. In a follow-up manuscript, Levi et al describe the clinical outcomes of this patient cohort (13). All 14 patients were American Spinal Injury Association and International Medical Society of Paraplegia Impairment Scale (AIS) A on admission. 8/14 patients remained so, but 3 improved to B, 2 to C and one patient had dramatic improvement to AIS D. Importantly, none of the patients worsened. A control group of patients only had 3/14 patients improve AIS grade compared with the six in the hypothermia group, a non-statistically significant difference. While the low number of patients, strict inclusion criteria, observational nature of study and use of an historical control may temper enthusiasm for these results, they are nonetheless intriguing and provide an excellent basis for developing future studies.

As mentioned previously, medical therapies for acute spinal cord injury are extremely limited. However, with future study, perhaps therapeutic hypothermia's role in treating the 11,000-12,000 spinal cord injury patients per year in the United States can further be defined (14).

3. Therapeutic hypothermia for intracerebral hemmorhage

Intracerebral hemorrhage (ICH) accounts for approximately 10% of all cerebral vascular accidents in the United States and carries a mortality rate of up to 50% (15,16). Options for medical therapy are extremely limited and are primarily focused on supportive therapy (17). Mayer et al investigated the potential use of rFVIIa for improving outcome and established that this therapy may in fact improve hematoma volume, but its impact on outcomes was limited (18). Hematoma volume & growth does correlate with various outcome measures (19-21), but so does perihemorrhagic edema (22-25). ICH is associated with secondary injury characteristics that are similar to ischemia and ischemia-reperfusion, including blood-brain barrier disruption, inflammation and edema. The edema progresses through three phases related initially to hydrostatic forces & clot retraction, then activation of the coagulation cascade and thrombin formation and later, via RBC lysis and hemoglobin-induced neuronal toxicity (26). This edema – termed *perihemorrhagic edema* – has been associated with poor outcomes (22, 23, 25). Data from animal models of ICH suggest that hypothermia can improve these injurious processes, but not outcomes (27-33).

There is a suggestion that the application of therapeutic hypothermia may be beneficial in preventing the progression of periphemorrhagic edema and improving outcomes in patients who suffer intracranial hemorrhage (34). In a pilot study by Kollmar et al, hypothermia was determined to be safe as well as potentially provide a positive effect on ICH perihemorrhagic edema (25). This was a comparison of 12 patients w/ supratentorial ICH >25mL in volume cooled with an intravascular cooling device to 33 degrees C with 12 historical controls. Amongst the control cohort, there were more patients with uncontrolled intracranial hypertension, perihemorrhagic edema progression and death. In a followup study by the same group, Staykov et al described similar findings with 25 patients with large ICH as compared with an historical control group (35). Again, perihemorrhagic edema remained mostly unchanged in the hypothermia group, but steadily increased in the historical control group, with a statistically significant difference in perihemorrhagic edema volume. This difference was also associated with a suggestion of mortality difference, but with such a small sample size it was not statistically significant. The mortality rate was 8.3% in the hypothermia cohort, 16.7% in the control group at 3 months and 28% vs 44% at one year. There is a prospective, multicenter, randomized controlled phase II trial currently underway to more formally evaluate this question using a similar protocol (36).

4. Therapeutic Hypothermia for Subarachnoid Hemorrhage

As in all neurocritical care related illnesses, fever control may be important for minimizing secondary injury (37). In subarachnoid hemorrhage, this is particularly true. As many as 72% of all SAH patients may experience fever (38). Infection should always be ruled out and treated aggressively (39); however, the fever needs to be controlled whether it is secondary to infection or not. Fever in SAH is strongly linked to poor outcome and increased length of stay (40), as well as vasospasm (41, 42), ischemic injury (43), cerebral edema and worsened intracranial hypertension (44). Even a single episode of fever has been associated with poorer outcomes. However, one can only definitively say that fever is *associated* with worsened outcomes, it may not be *causative*. In other words, it may simply be a marker of bad outcomes (45).

Whether fever is simply a marker for bad outcomes or something more, there is a suggestion that controlling fever may actually be neuroprotective. Oddo et al demonstrated that induced normothermia in 18 SAH patients resulted in a lower lactate-pyruvate ratio, fewer metabolic crises and lower ICP (46). But what about therapeutic hypothermia as a primary treatment modality – not just for fever control? Mild hypothermia has been shown to decrease cytotoxic edema, lactate accumulation and improve the metabolic stress response to SAH in rats (47). It has also been shown to lower ICP and improve outcomes in rats, including decreased neurologic deficits (48). In a dog model of SAH, therapeutic hypothermia decreased cerebral vasospasm, possibly by decreasing the rise in endothelin-1 and lessening the decrease of NO in CSF and the blood (49). In patients with SAH treated with therapeutic hypothermia, Kawamura used PET scans to demonstrate that hypothermia did decrease cerebral blood flow and oxygen metabolic rate (50). Seule et al. treated 100 patients with SAH who developed intracranial hypertension, symptomatic cerebral vasospasm or both, with mild therapeutic hypothermia (51). The majority of these patients had poor-grade SAH. 90 patients were evaluated at follow-up, 32 (35.6%) had survived with good neurologic outcome (Glasgow Outcome Scale 4 or 5) and 43 (47.8%) died. Side effects were common, including electrolyte disorders, pneumonia, thrombocytopenia and septic shock. From this study, the authors conclude that therapeutic hypothermia is a viable "last-resort option", but side effects are common and potentially severe.

One of those common side effects of this therapy, shivering, can be detrimental to patients. Similar to any condition for which therapeutic hypothermia is employed, shivering should be avoided if possible and treated aggressively if present. Shivering has been associated with higher oxygen consumption, reduced PbtO2, higher ICP and lower CPP and higher resting energy expenditure (52-54). A substudy of the Intraoperative Hypothermia Aneurysm Surgery Trial revealed that bradycardia, a common and expected side effect of hypothermia, was associated with a higher 3-month mortality rate after SAH. "Relative tachycardia" and nonspecific ST-T wave changes, also common with hypothermia therapy, were also associated with a mortality difference. The implications of these findings are not clear, but should be kept in mind when using this therapeutic approach (55).

5. Conclusion

Therapeutic hypothermia has already been shown to have a positive impact on survival and neurologic outcome for survivors of out-of-hospital cardiac arrest (2, 3). That benefit likely is related to hypothermia's impact on the multiple mechanisms of secondary brain injury. There is certainly potential for therapeutic hypothermia to reduce the secondary injury that results from brain and spinal cord injury as well. Many animal studies, but to this point only limited clinical studies, have suggested such an effect in treating patients that have suffered spinal cord injury, intracerebral hemorrhage or subarachnoid hemorrhage. Fortunately, the technology available to help us achieve and maintain the goals of targeted temperature management has made it easier to do so. The availability of that technology and increasing familiarity with its use will only serve to help investigators understand the potential impact of this therapy in brain and spinal cord injury. Medical therapy for these conditions is limited. Hopefully, future studies will clarify the potential role of therapeutic hypothermia in improving outcomes for these potentially devastating conditions.

Author details

David E. Tannehill

Department of Critical Care Medicine, Mercy Hospital, St. Louis, USA

6. References

[1] Polderman, Kees H. Mechanisms of action, physiological effects, and complications of hypothermia. Critical Care Medicine. 37(7):S186-S202, July 2009.

[2] Bernard, SA, Gray TW, Buist MD, Jones BM, Silvester W, Gutteridge G, Smith,K. Treatment of comatose survivors of out-of-hospital cardiac arrest with induced hypothermia. NEJM 346, 557-563.

[3] The Hypothermia After Cardiac Arrest Study Group. Mild Therapeutic Hypothermia to Improve the Neurologic Outcome after Cardiac Arrest. NEJM 346(8): 549-556.

[4] Kelly DL Jr, Lassiter KR, Calogero JA, et al. Effects of local hypothermia and tissue oxygenation studies in experimental paraplegia. J Neurosurg 1970;33:554-563.

[5] Demian YK, White RJ, Yashon D, et al. Anaesthesia for laminectomy and localized cord cooling in acute cervical spine injury. Report of three cases. Br J Anaesth 1971;43:973-9.

[6] Bricolo A, Ore GD, Da Pian R, et al. Local cooling in spinal cord injury. Surg Neurol 1976;6:101-106.

[7] Hansebout RR, Kuchner EF. Effects of local hypothermia and of steroids upon recovery from experimental spinal cord compression injury. Surg Neurol 1975;4:531-536.

[8] Kuchner EF, Hansebout RR. Combined steroid and hypothermia treatment of experimental spinal cord injury. Surg Neurol 1976;6L371-376.

[9] Dietrich, DW. Therapeutic hypothermia for spinal cord injury. Crit Care Med 2009; 37(Suppl.):S238-242.

[10] Dietrich DW, Levi AD, Wang M, Green B. Hypothermic treatment for acute spinal cord injury. Neurotherapeutics 2011(8):229-239.

[11] Cappuccino A, Bisson LJ, Carpenter B, et al. The use of systemic hypothermia for the treatment of an acute spinal cord injury in a professional football player. Spine (Phil Pa 1976). 2010 Jan 15;35(2):E57-62.

[12] Levi AD, Green BA, Wang M, et al. Clinical Application of Modest Hypothermia after Spinal Cord Injury. J Neurotrauma 2009; 26:407-415.

[13] Levi AD, Casella G, Green BA, et al. Clinical outcomes using modest intravascular hypothermia after acute cervical spinal cord injury. Neurosurgery 2010; 66:670-77.

[14] National Spinal Cord Injury Statistical Center. Spinal Cord Injury Facts and Figures at a Glance. Birmingham, Alabama: National Spinal Cord Injury Statistical Center, University of Alabama, 2010.

[15] Gebel, JM, Broderick JP. Intracerebral hemorrhage. Neurol Clin 2000; 18(2):419-438.

[16] Flaherty ML, et al. Long-term mortality after intracerebral hemorrhage. Neurology 2006;66(8):1182-1186.

[17] Broderick J, Connolly S, Feldmann E, et al. Guidelines for the management of spontaneous intracerebral hemorrhage in adults: 2007 update: a guideline from the American Heart Association/American Stroke Association Stroke Council, High Blood Pressure Research Council, and the Quality of Care and Outcomes in Research Interdisciplinary Working Group. Stroke 2007;38(6):2001-2023.

[18] Mayer SA, Brun NC, Begtrup K, et al. Efficacy and safety of recombinant activated factor VII for acute intracerebral hemorrhage. N Engl J Med. 2008 May 15;358(20):2127-37.

[19] Brott T, Broderick J, Kothari R, et al. Early hemorrhage growth in patients with intracerebral hemorrhage. Stroke. 1997 Jan;28(1):1-5.

[20] Davis SM, Broderick J, Hennerici M, et al. Hematoma growth is a determinant of mortality and poor outcome after intracerebral hemorrhage. Neurology. 2006 Apr 25;66(8):1175-81.

[21] Hemphill JC, Bonovich DC, Besmertis L, et al. The ICH score: a simple, reliable grading scale for intracerebral hemorrhage. Stroke. 2001;32:891-897.

[22] Zazulia AR, Diringer MN, Derdeyn CP, et al. Progression of mass effect after intracerebral hemorrhage. Stroke 1999;30:1167-1173.

[23] Fernandes HM, Siddique S, Banister K, et al. Continuous monitoring of ICP and CPP following ICH and its relationship to clinical, radiological and surgical parameters. Acta Neurochir Suppl 2000;76:463-66.

[24] Gebel JM, Jauch EC, Brott TG, et al. Relative edema volume is a predictor of outcome in patients with hyperacute spontaneous intracerebral hemorrhage. Stroke. 2002 Nov;33(11):2636-41.

[25] Kollmar R, Staykov D, Dorfler A, et al. Hypothermia reduces perihemorrhagic edema after intracerebral hemorrhage. Stroke 2010;41:1684-1689.

[26] Xi, G, Keep, RF, Hoff, JT. Mechanisms of brain injury after intracerebral haemorrhage. Lancet Neurol. 2006;5:53-63.

[27] Kawai, N, Kawanishi, M, Okauchi, M, et al. Effects of hypothermia on thrombin-induced brain edema formation. Brain Res. 2001;895:50-58.

[28] Fingas, M, Clark, DL, Colbourne, F. The effecs of selective brain hypothermia on intracerebral hemorrhage in rats. Exp. Neurol 2007;208:277-284.

[29] Kawanishi, M, Kawai, N, Nakamura, T, et al. Effect of delayed mild brain hypothermia on edema formation after intracerebral hemorrhage in rats. J Stroke Cerebrovasc Dis. 2008;17:187-195.

[30] MacLellan, CL, Auriat, AM, McGie, SC, et al. Gauging recovery after hemorrhagic stroke in rats: implications for cytoprotection studies. J Cereb Blood Flow Metab. 2006;26:1031-1042.

[31] MacLellan, CL, Davies LM, Fingas, MS, et al. The influence of hypothermia on outcome after intracerebral hemorrhage in rats. Stroke. 2006;37:1266-1270.

[32] Wagner, KR, Beiler, S, Beiler, C, et al. Delayed profound local brain hypothermia markedly reduces interleukin-1 beta gene expression and vasogenic edema development in a porcine model of intracerebral hemorrhage. Acta Neurochir. 2006;Suppl (96):177-182.

[33] Fingas, M, Penner, M, Silasi, G, et al. Treatment of intracerebral hemorrhage in rats with 12h, 3 days and 6 days of selective brain hypothermia. Exp Neurol. 2009;219:156-162.

[34] Feng, H, Shi, D, Wang, D, et al. Effect of local mild hypothermia on treatment of acute intracerebral hemorrhage, a clinical study. Zhounghua Yi Xue Za Zhi 2002;(82):1622-1624.

[35] Staykov D, Wagner I, Volbers B, et al. Mild Prolonged Hypothermia for Large Intracerebral Hemorrhage. Neurocrit Care. Published online August 3, 2012.

[36] Kollmar R, Juettler E, Huttner H, et al. Cooling in intracerebral hemorrhage (CINCH) trial: protocol of a randomized German-Austrian clinical trial. Int J Stroke. 2012;Feb;7(2):168-172.

[37] Badjiatia N. Hyperthermia and fever control in brain injury. Crit Care Med. 2009;37:S250-7.

[38] Scaravelli V, Tinchero G, Citerio G, et al. Fever Management in SAH. Neurocrit Care. 2011;15:287-294.

[39] O'Grady NP, Barie PS, Bartlett JG, et al. Guidelines for evaluation of new fever in critically ill adult patients: 2008 update from the American college of critical care medicine and the infectious disease society of America. Crit Care Med. 2008;36:1330-49.

[40] Diringer MN, Reaven NL, Funk SE, et al. Elevated body temperature independently contributes to increased length of stay in neurologic intensive care unit patients. Crit Care Med. 2004;32:1489-95.

[41] Wartenberg KE, Schmidt JM, Claassen J, et al. Impact of medical complications on outcoe after subarachnoid hemorrhage. Crit Care Med 2006;34:617-23.

[42] Oliveira-Filho J, Ezzeddine MA, Segal AZ. Fever in subarachnoid hemorrhage: relationship to vasospasm and outcome. Neurology. 2001;56:1299-304.

[43] Ginsberg MD, Busto R. combating hyperthermia in acute stroke: a significant clinical concern. Stroke. 1998;29:529-34.

[44] Rossi S, Zanier ER, Mauri I, et al. Brain temperature, body core temperature, and intracranial pressure in acute cerebral damage. J Neurol Neurosurg Psychiatry. 2001;71:448-54.

[45] Todd MM, Hindman BJ, Clarke WR, et al. Perioperative fever and outcome in surgical patients with aneursymal subarachnoid hemorrhage. Neurosurgery. 2009; May; 64(5):897-908.

[46] Oddo M, Frangos S, Milby A, et al. Induced normothermia attenuates cerebral metabolic distress in patients with aneurismal subarachnoid hemorrhage and refractory fever. Stroke. 2009;40:1913-6.

[47] Schubert et al. Hypothermia reduces cytotoxic edema and metabolic alterations during the acute phase of massive SAH: a diffusion weighted imaging and spectroscopy study in rats. J Neurotrauma 2008;Jul;25(7):841-52.

[48] Torok E, Klopotowksi M, Trabold R, et al. Mild hypothermia (33 degrees C) reduces intracranial hypertension and improves functional outcome after subarachnoid hemorrhage in rats. Neurosurgery. 2009;Aug;65(2):352-9.

[49] Wang Zp, Chen HS, Wang FX. Influence of plasma and cerebrospinal fluid levels of ednothelin-1 and NO in reducing cerebral vasospasm after subarachnoid hemorrhage during treatment with mild hypothermia, in a dog model. Cell Biochem Biophys. 2011;Sep;61(1):137-43.

[50] Kawamura S, Suzuki A, Hadeishi H, et al. Cerebral blood flow and oxygen metabolism during mild hypothermia in patients with subarachnoid haemorrhage. Acta Neurochir. 2000;142(10):1117-21.

[51] Seule MA, Muroi C, Mink S, et al. Therapeutic hypothermia in patients with aneurismal subarachonoid hemorrhage, refractory intracranial hypertension, or cerebral vasospasm. Neurosurgery 2009;Jan;64(1):86-92.

[52] Hata JS, Shelsky CR, Hindman BJ, et al. A prospective, observational clinical trial of fever reduction to reuce systemic oxygen consumption in the setting of acute brain injury. Neurocrit Care. 2008;9:37-44.

[53] Oddo M, Frangos S, Maloney-Wilensky E, et al. Effect of shivering on brain tissue oxygenation during induced normothermia in patients with severe brain injury. Neurocrit Care. 2009;12:10-6.

[54] Badjiatia N, Strongilis E, Gordon E, et al. Metabolic impact of shivering during therapeutic temperature modulation: the Bedside Shivering Assessment Scale. Stroke. 2008;Dec 39(12):3242-7.

[55] Coghlan LA, Hindman BJ, Bayman EO, et al. Independent associations between electrocardiographic abnormalitieis and outcomes in patients with aneurismal subarachnoid hemorrhage: findings from the introperative hypothermia aneurysm surgery trial. Stroke. 2009;Feb;40(2):412-8.

[56] Qureshi A, Mendelow AD, Hanley DF. Intracerebral haemorrhage. Lancet. 2009;373:1632-44.

[57] Staykov, D, Wagner I, Volbers B, et al. Natural course of perihemorrhagic edema after intracerebral hemorrhage. Stroke. 2011;42:2625-9.

[58] Staykov D, Schwab S, Dorfler A, Kollmer R. Hypothermia Reduces Perihemorrhagic Edema After Intracerebral Hemorrhage: But Does it Influence Functional Outcome and Mortality? Therapeutic Hypothermia and Temperature Management. 2011;1:(2):105-106.

[59] Xi, G, Keep RF, Hoff, JT. Pathophysiology of brain edema formation. Neurosurg Clin N Am. 2002;13:371-83.

Section 4

Therapeutic Hypothermia- Traumatic Brain Injury/Intracranial Hypertension

Chapter 6

Therapeutic Hypothermia in Traumatic Brain Injury

Farid Sadaka, Christopher Veremakis, Rekha Lakshmanan and Ashok Palagiri

Additional information is available at the end of the chapter

http://dx.doi.org/10.5772/48818

1. Introduction

Traumatic brain injury (TBI) is a major source of death and severe disability worldwide. In the USA alone, this type of injury causes 290,000 hospital admissions, 51,000 deaths, and 80,000 permanently disabled survivors [1,2]. Intracranial hypertension develops commonly in acute brain injury related to trauma [3,4]. Raised Intracranial pressure (ICP) is an important predictor of mortality in patients with severe TBI, and aggressive treatment of elevated ICP has been shown to reduce mortality and improve outcome [4-11]. Guidelines for the Management of Severe TBI, published in the Journal of Neurotrauma in 2007 [12] make a Level II recommendation that ICP should be monitored in all salvageable patients with a severe TBI (Glasgow Coma Scale [GCS] score of 3–8 after resuscitation) and an abnormal computed tomography (CT) scan. ICP monitoring is also recommended in patients with severe TBI and a normal CT scan if two or more of the following features are noted at admission: age over 40 years, unilateral or bilateral motor posturing, or systolic blood pressure < 90 mm Hg (Level III recommendation). Furthermore, ICP should be maintained less than 20 mmHg and cerebral perfusion pressure (CPP) between 50 and 70 mmHg (Level III).

As in ischemia –reperfusion injuries, the acute post-injury period in TBI is characterized by several pathophysiologic processes that start in the minutes to hours following injury and may last for hours to days. These result in further neuronal injury and are termed the secondary injury. Cellular mechanisms of secondary injury include all of the following: apoptosis, mitochondrial dysfunction, excitotoxicity, disruption in ATP metabolism, disruption in calcium homeostasis, increase in inflammatory mediators and cells, free radical formation, DNA damage, blood-brain barrier disruption, brain glucose utilization disruption, microcirculatory dysfunction and microvascular thrombosis [13-50]. All of these processes are temperature dependent; they are all aggravated by fever and inhibited by hypothermia [13-50]. In addition, several studies have shown that development of fever following TBI is closely linked to intracranial hypertension and worsened outcome [51-53].

Clinical trials of hypothermia and temperature management for severe traumatic brain injury are divided into trials in which hypothermia is used to treat elevated intracranial pressure and those in which hypothermia is intended as a neuroprotectant, irrespective of intracranial pressure. In this article, we will review the current clinical evidence behind therapeutic hypothermia for the treatment of intracranial hypertension (ICH) in severe TBI patients, as well as therapeutic hypothermia as a neuroprotectant in severe TBI.

2. Methods

We queried the Medline database with the MeSH terms "Hypothermia, induced," "Fever", "Intracranial Hypertension", and "Traumatic Brain Injury" from 1993 till 2011. We utilized both PubMed and OVID to maximize database penetration. We searched the Cochrane Database of Systematic Reviews. We also hand searched bibliographies of relevant citations and reviews. Inclusion criteria were double-blind, placebo-controlled, randomized controlled trials (RCTs), observational studies or meta-analysesof therapeutic hypothermia for TBI patients in which ICPs are monitored.We limited the search to human literature; We did not limit language, but we extracted studies that involved only adult subjects excluding studies on the pediatric population. Information extracted included number of patients, ICP, length of cooling, length of re-warming, outcome, complications, methods used to control ICP and the quality of each study. We reviewed the literature pertaining to pathophysiology of Traumatic Brain Injury. We also reviewed the literature pertaining to major published guidelines in this area.

3. Intracranial hypertension in TBI

In comatose TBI patients with an abnormal CT scan, the incidence of ICH was 53–63% [75]. Patients with a normal CT scan at admission, on the other hand, had a relatively low incidence of ICH (13%). However, within the normal CT group, if patients demonstrated at least two of three adverse features (age over 40 years, unilateral or bilateral motor posturing, or systolic BP < 90 mm Hg); their risk of ICH was similar to that of patients with abnormal CT scans [75]. ICP is a strong predictor of outcome from severe TBI [5,6, 9,76-78]. Because of this, ethically a randomized trial of ICP monitoring with and without treatment is unlikely to be carried out. Similarly, a trial for treating or not treating systemic hypotension is not likely. Both hypotension and raised ICP are the leading causes of death in severe TBI. Furthermore, several studies have shown that patients who do not have ICH or who respond to ICP-lowering therapies have a lower mortality than those whose ICH does not respond to therapy [4-11, 79-82]. As a result, Guidelines for the Management of Severe TBI recommend that treatment should be initiated with ICP thresholds above 20 mm Hg (level II) as well as target a cerebral perfusion pressure (CPP) within the range of 50-70 (level III) [12]. Prevention and/or treatment of ICH is commonly accomplished by employing a

Reference	No. of patients	Length of cooling	ICP(norm)	ICP(Hypo)	Length of rewarming	Outcome	Complications of hypothermia
Shiozaki et al, 1993	33	48 hrs	35.4	25 (p < 0.01)	24 hrs	6 month survival(50 % vs 18 %, p<0.05) Death from uncontrolled ICH(31% vs 71 %, p<0.05)	No difference
Marion et al, 1993	40	24 hrs	ICP > 20 (25 %)	ICP > 20 (13 %) (p<0.001)	12 hrs	3 month good GOS (60 % vs 40 %, p < 0.24)	No difference
Marion et al, 1997	82	24 hrs	19.7	15.4 (p=0.01)	12 hrs	12 month good neurologic outcome (62 % vs 38 %, p=0.05)	Elevated PTT, decreased potassium
Jiang et al, 2000	87	3 - 14 days	29.6	18.9 (P < 0.01)	1°C/hr	1 yr good GOS (46.5 % vs 27.3 %, p < 0.05) 1 yr mortality (25.6 % vs 45.5 %, p < 0.05)	--
Clifton et al, 2001	392	47 hrs	ICP > 30 (59%)	ICP > 30 (41%) (p=0.02)	18 hrs (0.25°C/hr)	No difference	Hypotension, bradycardia
Polderman et al, 2001	41	n/a	36	15 (p < 0.01)	n/a	No difference	Hypomagnesemia, hypocalcemia, hypokalemia, hypophosphatemia
Polderman et al, 2002	136	4.8 days	37	< 20 (p < 0.01)	1°C/12hrs	6 m good GOS (15.7 % vs 9.7 %, p<0.02) Mortality (62 % vs 72 %, p<0.05)	arrythmias
Gal et al, 2002	30	72 hrs	18	12 (p=0.0007)	passive	6 m good GOS (87% vs 47%)	---
Zhi et al, 2003	396	1-7 days (mean = 62 hrs)	26.9	14.8 (p< 0.05)	16-20 hrs (1°C/4hrs)	6 m Good GOS(38.8% vs 19.7%, p<0.05) Mortality (25.7% vs 36.4%, p<0.05)	hypokalemia
Smrcka et al, 2005	72	72 hrs	Primary (18.9) Extracerebral (16.6)	Primary(10.8) (p < 0.0001) Extracerebral (13.2)(p =0.1)	passive	Primary(6 m GOS: p=0.44) Extracerebral (6 m GOS: 3 to 5 ,p= 0.0006) Total 6 m good GOS(85% vs 48.5%)	bradycardia
Qiu et al, 2005	86	3-5 days	24 hrs:32.6 48 hrs:34.8 72 hrs:31.8	27.3 (p <0.05) 29.4 (p <0.05) 26.4 (p <0.05)	Passive (up to 24 hrs)	2 yr good GOS (65% vs 37%, p<0.05) Mortality (25.6% vs 51.2%, p<0.05)	Pneumonia, thrombocytopenia
Jiang et al, 2006	215	2 days vs 5 days	28(2 day hypothermia)	18(5 day hypothermia)	1°C/hr	6 m good GOS(43.5% in 5 day group vs 29% in 2 day group, p < 0.05)	More rebound increase in ICP in 2 day group (p < 0.05) Pneumonia and arrhythmias (similar)
Qiu et al, 2007	80	4 days	24 hrs:25.8 48 hrs:25.9 72 hrs:24.6	23.5 (p=0.00) 24.6 (p=0.00) 22.5(p=0.003)	Passive(10- 24 hrs)	1 yr good neurologic outcome GOS (70% vs 47.5%, p=0.041)	Pneumonia, thrombocytopenia

GOS = Glascow Outcome Score

Table 1. Effects of Hypothermia on intracranial pressure and outcome in patients with severe Traumatic Brain Injury: Randomized Controlled Trials

progression of therapeutic approaches that are efficacious in controlling ICP and uniformly believed to be easily applied with minimal or rare negative side effects. These measures include elevation of the head of the bed , avoiding hypotension, hypoxia, and hypercapnea or prolonged hypocapnea, intravenous sedation and analgesia, episodic administration of hyperosmolar agents (mannitol, hypertonic saline), and CSF drainage [12]. Reviewing the evidence behind all these aforementioned therapies is beyond the scope of this review, but the evidence of efficacy for all of these treatments is variable at best. They are recommended not so much because there is clear-cut proof of morbidity or mortality benefit but because they are deemed treatments without significant downside.

4. Therapeutic hypothermia for ICP control

We identified a total of 18 studies involving hypothermia for control of ICP; 13 were randomized clinical trials and 5 were observational studies as shown in tables 1 and 2 respectively [54, 58-74]. In all studies, the patient populations were comprised of TBI patients with GCS < 9 and an abnormal CT scan. ICP monitors were inserted in all patients to measure ICP. Individual study sizes ranged from 9 to 396 patients; a total of 1,773 patients were included in this review. Only three studies were multicenter [54,72,74]. The goals of therapy were stabilization or improvement of the patient's neurological condition, and maintenance of an ICP of 20 mmHg or less (normal value in healthy subjects: ≤15 mmHg) and a cerebral perfusion pressure (CPP = MAP– ICP) of 60 mmHg or more or 70 mmHg or more. In patients with ICP higher than 20 mmHg, initial (standard) treatment included appropriate sedatives, narcotics, treatment with neuromuscular blockers (for ICP control and/or shivering) and administration of hyperosmolar therapy. Neurosurgical interventions were undertaken when necessary to evacuate subdural lesions or large intracerebral lesions [58, 61, 63, 64, 66-74]. In nine studies, there was no mention of the use barbiturates for ICP control [60, 62, 64, 68, 69, 71-74]. In five of the studies, therapeutic hypothermia was applied after elevated ICP failed to respond to adequate sedation, hyperosmolar therapy and barbiturates [58, 63, 65-67]. In the other four studies [54,59, 61,70], patients were randomized to hypothermia or normothermia irrespective of ICP, with the goal of studying hypothermia's role as a neuroprotectant (discussed below). ICP control was looked at as a secondary outcome in these four studies.

Target temperature (32^0C – 34 ^{0}C) was achieved very quickly in most studies. Therapeutic hypothermia was maintained from 24 hrs up to 14 days depending on the study protocols. Some studies achieved re-warming passively over 10- 24 hrs [67,70, 71,73], but most studies achieved slow active rewarming over 12- 24 hrs as shown in tables 1 and 2. In one study, hypothermia maintenance for five days was associated with less rebound ICH than hypothermia for two days [72]. Therapeutic hypothermia was effective in controlling ICH in all studies as shown in tables 1 and 2 and figure 1. In the 13 RCT, ICP in the therapeutic hypothermia group was always lower than ICP in the normothermia group, and this difference always reached statistical significance as evidenced in table 1 and figure 1. In the 5 observational studies, ICP during hypothermia was always lower then prior to inducing hypothermia; this difference also always reached statistical significance as shown in table 2. Therapeutic hypothermia also improved neurologic outcome and survival in eleven of the studies as can be seen in table 1.

Reference	No. of patients	Length of cooling	ICP(pre)	ICP(Hypo)	Length of rewarming	Outcome	Complications of hypothermia
Metz et al, 1996	10	25 hrs	24	14 (p< 0.05)	22 hrs	7 patients (good recovery) 1 patient (severe disability) 2 patients (dead)	Thrombocytopenia, decreased creatinine clearance, pancreatitis
Nara et al, 1998	9	n/a	20	12 (P < 0.05)	n/a	3 m good GOS (8/9= 88.8%)	n/a
Tateishi et al, 1998	9	20-118 hrs (mean=68 hrs)	24	15 (p < 0.05)	< 1ºC/6hrs	Good GOS 7/9	Infection, increase CRP, thrombocytopenia
Tokutomi et al, 2003	31	48 – 72 hrs	24	14 (p<0.0001)	n/a	6m Good GOS (19%) Mortality (48%)	pneumonia
Sahuquillo et al, 2009	24	155 hrs	23.8	16.8 (p < 0.001)	1ºC/day	6 month Neurologic outcome (Good: 29.2 %, moderate: 8.3 %)	arrythmias

GOS = Glascow Outcome Score

Table 2. Effects of Hypothermia on intracranial pressure and outcome in patients with severe Traumatic Brain Injury: Nonrandomized Observational Trials

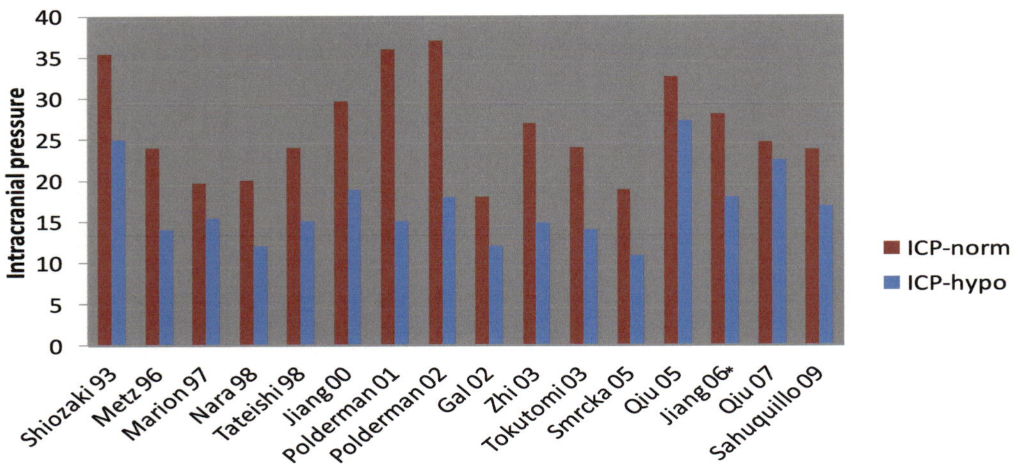

Reference: In Jiang 06, the comparison is between 2 days of hypothermia (red) and 5 days of hypothermia (blue)

Figure 1. Effect of Hypothermia on Intracranial Pressure (ICP).

5.Therapeutic hypothermia as a neuroprotectant

The premise of the use of TH as a neuroprotectant in TBI is based on the fact that early administration of TH could halt the secondary injury processes discussed above, and thus possibly improve outcome. We identified a total of 9 studies where TH is used as a neuroprotectant in TBI, 5 of the studies designed to deliver TH as a neuroprotectant [54-56,61,70], and 4 of the studies designed to deliver TH for neuroprotection and ICP control [48,64,72,73] (Table 3). In all studies, the patient populations were comprised of TBI patients with GCS < 9 and an abnormal CT scan. ICP monitors were inserted in all patients to measure ICP. Individual study sizes ranged from 26 to 392 patients. In the 4 studies designed to deliver hypothermia for ICP control and as a neuroprotectant, ICP in the TH group was always lower than ICP in the normothermia group, and this difference always reached statistical significance. Outcome was better in the hypothermia group in all of these 4 studies.

The 5 Trials designed with early administration of hypothermia for neuroprotection are described as such:

Marion et al in 1997 enrolled 82 patients of ages 16–75 years where patients assigned to hypothermia were cooled to 33⁰C a mean of 10 hours after injury, kept cool for 24 hours, and rewarmed over 24 hours [61]. At 1 year followup, 38 % of the patients in the hypothermia group and 62% of those in the normothermia group had poor outcomes (p = 0.05). The reported effect was exclusively in patients with admission GCS 5–7 [61]. Clifton in 2001 enrolled 392 patients ages 16–65 years with target temperature of 33⁰C reached by a little more than 8 hours after injury and maintained for 48 hours [54]. Rewarming was started at 48 hours irrespective of ICP, at a rate of 0.5⁰C every 2 hours. Outcome at 6 months was poor in 57% of patients in both groups. In subgroup analyses, adverse outcome was associated with hypothermia induction in patients older than 45 years of age, and better outcome was associated with maintenance of hypothermia in patients who were already hypothermic (<35⁰C) on admission [54]. In this study, TH was started fairly late and cooling was slow (average time to target temperature >8 h), and there were problems with hypotension, hypovolemia, electrolytes, and hyperglycaemia. Hypotensive episodes lasting for more than 2 h occurred three times more frequently in the hypothermia group than in the control group. Since even very brief episodes of hypotension or hypovolemia can adversely affect outcome in TBI, these problems might have greatly affected the results of this trial. In 2001, Shiozaki et al enrolled 91 patients who did not have elevated ICP in a study comparing the effect of 48 hours of hypothermia with normothermia [55]. There was no difference in outcome, with 53% of patients in the hypothermia group and 51% of patients in the normothermia group having poor outcomes. The incidences of pneumonia, meningitis, thrombocytopenia, leukocytopenia, hypernatremia, hypokalemia, and hyperamylasemia were higher in the hypothermia than in the normothermia group [55]. In 2005, Smrcka et al. reported a study of 72 patients in whom hypothermia maintained for 72 hours was compared to normothermia [70]. There was no difference in outcome between the two groups. However, patients treated with hypothermia with extracerebral hematomas but not diffuse brain injury had a significantly better Glasgow Outcome Score at 6 months than patients treated at normothermia [70]. In 2011, Clifton et al. started hypothermia in transit to or in the emergency department in a study enrolling 97 patients with TBI [56]. Hypothermia was maintained for 48 hours and patients rewarmed at 0.5⁰C every 2 hours. A protocol of aggressive fluid expansion during rewarming and low dose morphine was used to prevent the hypotension that had complicated use of hypothermia in the group's first study (above). Overall, there was no improvement in outcome at 6 months, but there was a difference in outcomes of patients with diffuse brain injury and those with evacuated hematomas (p = 0.001). Fewer patients with evacuated hematomas treated with hypothermia had poor outcomes (hypothermia - 33%, normothermia - 69%, p = 0.02), whereas more patients with diffuse brain injury treated with hypothermia had poor outcomes (hypothermia - 70%, normothermia - 50%, p = 0.09). Patients treated with hypothermia had a higher number of total episodes of elevated ICP, especially during rewarming [56]. Again, in this study, hypothermia was maintained for a fixed duration of only 48 hrs, and ICP elevations mainly occurred during and after rewarming. In addition, there were deviations from the protocol in this study, for example the decision to advance the interim analysis, and thus the enrollment of a smaller number of patients than planned.

Reference	No. of patients	ICP control	Neuro-protection	Length of cooling	Outcome
[redacted]					
Abiki et al,2000	26	yes	yes	3 – 5 days	positive
Jiang et al,2000	87	yes	yes	3-14 days	positive
Jiang et al,2006	215	yes	yes	2 or 5 days	positive
Qui et al, 2007	80	Yes	Yes	4 days	positive
Marion et al,1997	82		Yes	24 hours	positive
Clifton et al,2001	392		Yes	48 hours	No improvement
Shiazaki et al,2001	91		Yes	48 hours	No improvement
Smrcka et al,2005	72		Yes	72 hours	No improvement
Clifton et al,2011	97		Yes	48 hours	No improvement

Table 3. Studies where Therapeutic Hypothermia is used as a neuroprotectant.

6. Side effects of therapeutic hypothermia in TBI

Complications from hypothermia included electrolyte imbalances, increase in incidence of infections, thrombocytopenia, coagulopathy, arrhythmias (especially bradycardia), pancreatitis, and rebound ICH (during re-warming) as presented in tables 1 & 2. Particular consideration should be given to the rate of rewarming. In one extensive review [84], Povlishock et al showed that posttraumatic hypothermia followed by slow rewarming appeared to provide maximal protection in terms of traumatically induced axonal damage, microvascular damage and dysfunction, contusional expansion, intracranial hypertension, and neurocognitive recovery. In contrast, hypothermia followed by rapid rewarming not only reversed the protective effects associated with hypothermic intervention, but exacerbated the traumatically induced pathology and its neurologic consequences. Povlishock's review concluded that the rate of posthypothermic rewarming is an important variable in assuring maximal efficacy following the use of hypothermic intervention. Two meta-analyses [12, 85] as well showed that duration >48 h and slow rewarming were associated with improved outcome.

7. Discussion

Multiple trials, albeit observational or small single center randomized controlled studies, show that mild to moderate hypothermia consistently lowers high ICP in severe TBI patients as shown in figure 1. It is an accepted premise in the care of severe TBI patients that control of ICP improves survival and possibly neurologic outcome. It follows therefore that induced hypothermia in patients with poorly controlled ICP may be a reasonable therapeutic strategy when routine sedation, analgesia and neuromuscular paralysis fail. This benefit would be relevant regardless of any cellular or metabolic neuroprotective effect. Indeed, the additional potential neuroprotective benefits suggest that therapeutic hypothermia if without negative side effects should be implemented as a part of routine ICP control rather than as rescue therapy. It is puzzling why barbiturates with the well-known negative side effects are recommended while hypothermia with its known efficacy in controlling ICH is not. The reasons for this may be the relative inexperience with TH, complexity of TH implementation, concerns for adverse reactions, and the need for sophisticated technology [86,87]. In 2002, studies have indicated that TH with a reduction of body core temperature (T) to 33 °C over 12 to 24 hours has improved survival and neurologic outcome in cardiac arrest patients [88, 89]. A meta-analysis showed that therapeutic hypothermia for cardiac arrest patients was associated with a risk ratio of 1.68 (95% CI, 1.29-2.07) favoring a good neurologic outcome when compared with normothermia [90]. The number needed to treat (NNT) to generate one favorable neurological recovery was 6. Subsequently, the International Liaison Committee on Resuscitation [91] and the American Heart Association [92] recommended the use of TH after sudden cardiac arrest. As a result, intensivists and neurointensivists have become much more familiar with the methodology (following cardiac arrest) so that the process is now familiar. And with appropriate hypothermia protocols, order sets, and education programs, mild hypothermia can be accomplished with very few side effects. It is important to note, however, that there are important differences between short duration hypothermia following cardiac arrest and long term hypothermia in TBI patients with ICH who frequently also have extracranial injuries and extra attention to the above mentioned side effects should be applied. Hypothermia should no longer be viewed as avant guard or dangerous, and we believe that it should take the place of barbiturates as the best modality for refractory ICH. Indeed, there is an argument, pending large scale studies, to consider it an extension of standard treatment. Pending large multicenter, randomized, controlled trials evaluating the effect of hypothermia on ICP control and outcome, the available data suggests that therapeutic hypothermia deserves at least a level II evidence recommendation for the treatment of refractory ICH.

As for trials classified as designed for neuroprotection, although single-center studies were encouraging, multicenter trials with early administration of hypothermia for a defined period of time irrespective of ICP have almost uniformly been negative except maybe for patients undergoing craniotomy for hematoma evacuations. However, hypothermia was maintained for a fixed duration of only 48 hrs, and ICP elevations mainly occurred during and after rewarming. These results suggest that a period of 48 hours of hypothermia may be too short to have a beneficial effect on outcome. A standardized one size fit all may be inappropriate. The rate of rewarming plays an important role as well as pointed above. The rebound increase in ICP during and after rewarming in these studies and the encouraging outcomes from the randomized studies that induced hypothermia early and continued it throughout the period of ICP point to the realization that individualizing the duration of hypothermia to fit a patient's ICP in future trials may be a better strategy than a predetermined period of hypothermia regardless of ICP. Another important finding is the differential effect of hypothermia in patients with surgical lesions versus those with diffuse injuries. This could be explained by the ability for volume expansion after surgery and thus less rebound ICP during and after rewarming. However, no final answer on this differential effect can be given at this stage, especially with the low number of patients studied so far. As a result, there is no reason to exclude patients with diffuse injury from future trials.

8. Conclusion

Preliminary evidence points to the effectiveness of mild to moderate therapeutic hypothermia in controlling ICH in severe TBI patients. The experience with induced hypothermia in the treatment of post cardiac arrest patients has demonstrated an acceptable safety profile when the modality is applied in specialized units by experienced personell according to a defined protocol. In addition, the above mentioned studies of therapeutic hypothermia in TBI patients show that the adverse effects of hypothermia are reasonable and managable when hypothermia is done in specialized and experienced ICUs. Pending results from large multicenter studies evaluating the effect of therapeutic hypothermia on ICH and outcome, therapeutic hypothermia should be included as a therapeutic option to control ICP in severe TBI patients. The most challenging issue appears to be rebound ICP during re-warming. We suggest that re-warming only be considered if the patient's ICP is stable and <20mmHg for at least 48 hours, and, thereafter implemented at a rate not faster than 0.25°C per hour. As for future of hypothermia as a neuroprotectant in TBI patients irrespective of ICP, Individualizing the duration of hypothermia to fit a patient's ICP in future trials is a better strategy than a predetermined period of hypothermia regardless of ICP. Design of these trials should also consider both the mechanism being tested and the differential effect between patients with evacuated hematomas and those with diffuse brain injury.

Author details

Farid Sadaka, Christopher Veremakis, Rekha Lakshmanan and Ashok Palagiri
Mercy Hospital St Louis/St Louis University,
Critical Care Medicine/Neurocritical Care, St Louis, USA

Acknowledgement

No additional acknowledgements.

Conflicts of Interest

The authors report no conflicts of interest.

All authors declare that No competing financial interests exist.

All authors report that no potential conflicts of interest exist with any companies/ organizations whose products or services may be discussed in this article.

9. References

[1] Dombovy ML, Olek AC (1997) Recovery and rehabilitation following traumatic brain injury. Brain Inj. 11(5):305-18.

[2] Rutland-Brown W, Langlois JA, Thomas KE, Xi YL (2006) Incidence of traumatic brain injury in the United States, 2003. J Head Trauma Rehabil 21: 544 - 48.

[3] Miller JD, Becker DP, Ward JD, Sullivan HG, Adams WE, Rosner MJ (1977) Significance of intracranial hypertension in severe head injury. J Neurosurg 47:503–516.

[4] Miller JD, Dearden NM, Piper IR, Chan KH (1992) Control of intracranial pressure in patients with severe head injury. J Neurotrauma 9(suppl 1):S317–S326.

[5] Marmarou A, Anderson PL, Ward JD, Choi SC, Young HF (1991) Impact of ICP instability and hypotension on outcome in patients with severe head trauma. J Neurosurg 75(suppl):59–66.

[6] Ghajar J, Hariri RJ, Patterson RH (1993) Improved outcome from traumatic coma using only ventricular cerebrospinal fluid drainage for intracranial pressure control. Adv Neurosurg 21:173–177.

[7] Juul N, Morris GF, Marshall SB, Marshall LF (2000) Intracranial hypertension and cerebral perfusion pressure: influence on neurological deterioration and outcome in severe head injury. The Executive Committee of the International Selfotel Trial. J Neurosurg 92:1– 6.

[8] Steiner T, Ringleb P, Hacke W (2001) Treatment options for large hemispheric stroke. Neurology 57:S61–S68.

[9] Becker DP, Miller JD, Ward JD, Greenberg RP, Young HF, Sakalas R (1977) The outcome from severe head injury with early diagnosis and intensive management. J Neurosurg 47:491– 502.

[10] Qureshi AI, Geocadin RG, Suarez JI, Ulatowski JA (2000) Long-term outcome after medical reversal of transtentorial herniation in patients with supratentorial mass lesions. Crit Care Med 28:1556 –1564.

[11] Patel HC, Menon DK, Tebbs S, Hawker R, Hutchinson PJ, Kirkpatrick PJ (2002) Specialist neurocritical care and outcome from head injury. Intensive Care Med 28:547–553.

[12] Brain Trauma Foundation; American Association of Neurological Surgeons; Congress of Neurological Surgeons; Joint Section on Neurotrauma and Critical Care, AANS/CNS (2007) Guidelines for the management of severe traumatic brain injury. J Neurotrauma 24 (Suppl 1):1-117.

[13] Small DL, Morley P, Buchan AM (1999) Biology of ischemic cerebral cell death. Prog Cardiovasc Dis 42:185–207.

[14] Milde LN (1992) Clinical use of mild hypothermia for brain protection. A dream revisited. J Neurosurg Anesthesiol 4:211–215.

[15] Hagerdal M, Harp J, Nilsson L, Siesjö BK (1975) The effect of induced hypothermia upon oxygen consumption in the rat brain. J Neurochem 24:311–316.

[16] Povlishock JT, Buki A, Koiziumi H, Stone J, Okonkwo DO (1999) Initiating mechanisms involved in the pathobiology of traumatically induced axonal injury and interventions targeted at blunting their progression. Acta Neurochir Suppl (Wien) 73:15–20.

[17] Xu L, Yenari MA, Steinberg GK, Giffard RG (2002) Mild hypothermia reduces apoptosis of mouse neurons in vitro early in the cascade. J Cereb Blood Flow Metab 22:21–28.

[18] Liou AK, Clark RS, Henshall DC, Yin XM, Chen J (2003) To die or not to die for neurons in ischemia, traumatic brain injury and epilepsy: A review on the stress-activated signaling pathways and apoptotic pathways. Prog Neurobiol 69:103–142.

[19] Leker RR, Shohami E (2002) Cerebral ischemia and trauma—different etiologies yet similar mechanisms: Neuroprotective opportunities. Brain Res Brain Res Re 39: 55–73.

[20] Raghupathi R, Graham DI, McIntosh TK (2000) Apoptosis after traumatic brain injury. J Neurotrauma 17:927–938.

[21] Globus MY-T, Busto R, Lin B, Schnippering H, Ginsberg MD (1995) Detection of free radical activity during transient global ischemia and recirculation: Effects of intra-ischemic brain temperature modulation. J Neurochem 65:1250–1256.

[22] Siesjo BK, Bengtsson F, Grampp W, Theander S (1989) Calcium, excitotoxins, and neuronal death in brain. Ann NY Acad Sci 568: 234 –251.

[23] Auer RN (2001) Non-pharmacologic (physiologic) neuroprotection in the treatment of brain ischemia. Ann NY Acad Sci 939: 271–282.

[24] Dempsey RJ, Combs DJ, Maley ME, Cowen DE, Roy MW, Donaldson DL (1987) Moderate hypothermia reduces postischemic edema development and leukotriene production. Neurosurgery 21: 177–181.

[25] Globus MY-T, Alonso O, Dietrich WD, Busto R, Ginsberg MD (1995) Glutamate release and free radical production following brain injury: Effects of posttraumatic hypothermia. J Neurochem 65:1704–1711.

[26] Busto R, Dietrich WD, Globus MY, Valdés I, Scheinberg P, Ginsberg MD (1987) Small differences in intraischemic brain temperature critically determine the extent of ischemic neuronal injury. J Cereb Blood Flow Metab 7:729–738.

[27] Baker AJ, Zornow MH, Grafe MR, Scheller MS, Skilling SR, Smullin DH, Larson AA (1991) Hypothermia prevents ischemia-induced increases in hippocampal glycine concentrations in rabbits. Stroke 22: 666–673.

[28] Kaibara T, Sutherland GR, Colbourne F, Tyson RL (1999) Hypothermia: Depression of tricarboxylic acid cycle flux and evidence for pentose phosphate shunt upregulation. J Neurosurg 90:339–347.

[29] Takata K, Takeda Y, Morita K (2005) Effects of hypothermia for a short period on histological outcome and extracellular glutamate concentration during and after cardiac arrest in rats. Crit Care Med 33: 1340–1345.

[30] Dietrich WD, Chatzipanteli K, Vitarbo E, Wada K, Kinoshita K (2004) The role of inflammatory processes in the pathophysiology and treatment of brain and spinal cord trauma. Acta Neurochir Suppl 89:69–74.

[31] Schmidt OI, Heyde CE, Ertel W, Stahel PF (2005) Closed head injury—an inflammatory disease? Brain Res Brain Res Rev 48: 388–399.

[32] Aibiki M, Maekawa S, Ogura S, Kinoshita Y, Kawai N, Yokono S (1999) Effect of moderate hypothermia on systemic and internal jugular plasma IL-6 levels after traumatic brain injury in humans. J Neurotrauma 16:225–232.

[33] Kimura A, Sakurada S, Ohkuni H, Todome Y, Kurata K (2002) Moderate hypothermia delays proinflammatory cytokine production of human peripheral blood mononuclear cells. Crit Care Med 30:1499–1502.

[34] Suehiro E, Fujisawa H, Akimura T, Ishihara H, Kajiwara K, Kato S, Fujii M, Yamashita S, Maekawa T, Suzuki M (2004) Increased matrix metalloproteinase-9 in blood in association with activation of interleukin-6 after traumatic brain injury: Influence of hypothermic therapy. J Neurotrauma 21: 1706–1711.

[35] Novack TA, Dillon MC, Jackson WT (1996) Neurochemical mechanisms in brain injury and treatment: A review. J Clin Exp Neuropsychol 18:685–706.

[36] Raghupathi R, McIntosh TK (1998) Pharmacotherapy for traumatic brain injury: A review. Proc West Pharmacol Soc 41: 241–246.

[37] Smith SL, Hall ED (1996) Mild pre- and posttraumatic hypothermia attenuates blood–brain barrier damage following controlled cortical impact injury in the rat. J Neurotrauma 13:1–9.

[38] Jurkovich GJ, Pitt RM, Curreri PW, Granger DN (1988) Hypothermia prevents increased capillary permeability following ischemia–reperfusion injury. J Surg Res 44:514–521.

[39] Chatauret N, Zwingmann C, Rose C, Leibfritz D, Butterworth RF(2003) Effects of hypothermia on brain glucose metabolism in acute liver failure: A H/C nuclear magnetic resonance study. Gastroenterology 125:815–824.

[40] Vaquero J, Blei AT (2005) Mild hypothermia for acute liver failure: A review of mechanisms of action. J Clin Gastroenterol 39: S147–S157.

[41] Soukup J, Zauner A, Doppenberg EM, Menzel M, Gilman C, Bullock R, Young HF (2002) Relationship between brain temperature, brain chemistry and oxygen delivery

after severe human head injury: The effect of mild hypothermia. Neurol Res 24: 161–168.

[42] Kimura T, Sako K, Tanaka K, Kusakabe M, Tanaka T, Nakada T (2002) Effect of mild hypothermia on energy state recovery following transient forebrain ischemia in the gerbil. Exp Brain Res 145:83–90.

[43] Bo¨ttiger BW, Motsch J, Bohrer H, Böker T, Aulmann M, Nawroth PP, Martin E (1995) Activation of blood coagulation after cardiac arrest is not balanced adequately by activation of endogenous fibrinolysis. Circulation 92:2572–2578.

[44] Gando S, Kameue T, Nanzaki S, Nakanishi Y (1997) Massive fibrin formation with consecutive impairment of fibrinolysis in patients with out-of-hospital cardiac arrest. Thromb Haemost 77:278–282.

[45] Michelson AD, MacGregor H, Barnard MR, Kestin AS, Rohrer MJ, Valeri CR (1994) Hypothermia-induced reversible platelet dysfunction. Thromb Haemost 71:633–640.

[46] Watts DD, Trask A, Soeken K, Perdue P, Dols S, Kaufmann C (1998) Hypothermic coagulopathy in trauma: Effect of varying levels of hypothermia on enzyme speed, platelet function, and fibrinolytic activity. J Trauma 44:846–854.

[47] Hsu CY, Halushka PV, Hogan EL, Banik NL, Lee WA, Perot PL Jr (1985) Alteration of thromboxane and prostacyclin levels in experimental spinal cord injury. Neurology 35:1003–1009.

[48] Aibiki M, Maekawa S, Yokono S (2000) Moderate hypothermia improves imbalances of thromboxane A2 and prostaglandin I2 production after traumatic brain injury in humans. Crit Care Med 28:3902–3906.

[49] Chen L, Piao Y, Zeng F, Lu M, Kuang Y, Ki X (2001) Moderate hypothermia therapy for patients with severe head injury. Chin J Traumatol 4:164–167.

[50] Schaller B, Graf R. Hypothermia and stroke (2003) The pathophysiological background. Pathophysiology 10:7–35.

[51] Rossi S, Zanier ER, Mauri I, Columbo A, Stocchetti N (2001) Brain temperature, body core temperature, and intracranial pressure in acute cerebral damage. J Neurol Neurosurg Psychiatry 71:448–454.

[52] Soukup J, Zauner A, Doppenberg EM, Menzel M, Gilman C, Young HF, Bullock R (2002) The importance of brain temperature in patients after severe head injury: relationship to intracranial pressure, cerebral perfusion pressure, cerebral blood flow, and outcome. J Neurotrauma 19:559–571.

[53] Diringer MN, Reaven NL, Funk SE, Uman GC (2004) Elevated body temperature independently contributes to increased length of stay in neurologic intensive care unit patients. Crit Care Med 32:1611–1612.

[54] Clifton GL, Miller ER, Choi SC, Levin HS, McCauley S, Smith KR Jr, Muizelaar JP, Wagner FC Jr, Marion DW, Luerssen TG, Chesnut RM, Schwartz M (2001) Lack of effect of induction of hypothermia after acute brain injury. N Engl J Med 344(8):556–63.

[55] Shiozaki T, Hayakata T, Taneda M, Nakajima Y, Hashiguchi N, Fujimi S, Nakamori Y, Tanaka H, Shimazu T, Sugimoto H (2001) A multicenter prospective randomized

induced trial of the efficacy of mild hypothermia for severely head injured patients with low intracranial pressure. Mild hypothermia study group in Japan. J Neurosurg 94(1):50–4.

[56] Clifton GL, Valadka A, Zygun D, Coffey CS, Drever P, Fourwinds S, Janis LS, Wilde E, Taylor P, Harshman K, Conley A, Puccio A, Levin HS, McCauley SR, Bucholz RD, Smith KR, Schmidt JH, Scott JN, Yonas H, Okonkwo DO (2011) Very early hypothermia induction in patients with severe brain injury (the National Acute Brain Injury Study: Hypothermia II): a randomised trial. The Lancet Neurology 10 (2): 131 – 139.

[57] Maas A, Stocchetti N (2011) Hypothermia and the complexity of trials in patients with traumatic brain injury. Lancet Neurology 10(2):111-3.

[58] Shiozaki T, Sugimoto H, Taneda M, Yoshida H, Iwai A, Yoshioka T, Sugimoto T (1993) Effect of mild hypothermia on uncontrollable intracranial hypertension after severe head injury. J Neurosurg 79(3):363-8.

[59] Marion DW, Obrist WD, Carlier PM, Penrod LE, Darby JM (1993) The use of moderate therapeutic hypothermia for patients with severe head injuries: a preliminary report. J Neurosurg 79: 354–62.

[60] Metz C, Holzschuh M, Bein T, Woertgen C, Frey A, Frey I, Taeger K, Brawanski A (1997) Moderate hypothermia in patients with severe head injury: cerebral and extracerebral effects. J Neurosurg 86(5):911-4.

[61] Marion DW, Penrod LE, Kelsey SF, Obrist WD, Kochanek PM, Palmer AM, Wisniewski SR, DeKosky ST (1997) Treatment of traumatic brain injury with moderate hypothermia. N Engl J Med 336: 540–46.

[62] Nara I, Shiogai T, Hara M, Saito I (1998) Comparative effects of hypothermia, barbiturate, and osmotherapy for cerebral oxygen metabolism, intracranial pressure, and cerebral perfusion pressure in patients with severe head injury. Acta Neurochir Suppl 71:22-6.

[63] Tateishi A, Soejima Y, Taira Y, Nakashima K, Fujisawa H, Tsuchida E, Maekawa T, Ito H (1998) Feasibility of the titration method of mild hypothermia in severely head-injured patients with intracranial hypertension. Neurosurgery 42(5):1065-9.

[64] Jiang J, Yu M, Zhu C (2000) Effect of long-term mild hypothermia therapy in patients with severe traumatic brain injury: 1-year follow-up review of 87 cases. J Neurosurg 93(4):546-9.

[65] Polderman KH, Peerdeman SM, Girbes AR (2001) Hypophosphatemia and hypomagnesemia induced by cooling in patients with severe head injury. J Neurosurg 94: 697–705.

[66] Polderman KH, Tjong Tjin Joe R, Peerdeman SM, Vandertop WP, Girbes AR (2002) Effects of therapeutic hypothermia on intracranial pressure and outcome in patients with severe head injury. Intensive Care Med 28: 1563–67.

[67] Gal R, Cundrle I, Zimova I, Smrcka M (2002) Mild hypothermia therapy for patients with severe brain injury. Clin Neurol Neurosurg 104: 318–21.

[68] Zhi D, Zhang S, Lin X (2003) Study on therapeutic mechanism and clinical effect of mild hypothermia in patients with severe head injury. Surg Neurol 59: 381–85.

[69] Tokutomi T, Morimoto K, Miyagi T, Yamaguchi S, Ishikawa K, Shigemori M (2003) Optimal temperature for the management of severe traumatic brain injury: effect of hypothermia on intracranial pressure, systemic and intracranial hemodynamics, and metabolism. Neurosurgery 52(1):102-11.

[70] Smrcka M, Vidlák M, Máca K, Smrcka V, Gál R (2005) The influence of mild hypothermia on ICP, CPP and outcome in patients with primary and secondary brain injury. Acta Neurochir Suppl 95: 273-5.

[71] Qiu WS, Liu WG, Shen H, Wang WM, Hang ZL, Zhang Y, Jiang SJ, Yang XF (2005) Therapeutic eff ect of mild hypothermia on severe traumatic head injury. Chin J Traumatol 8: 27–32.

[72] Jiang JY, Xu W, Li WP, Gao GY, Bao YH, Liang YM, Luo QZ (2006) Effect of long-term mild hypothermia or short-term mild hypothermia on outcome of patients with severe traumatic brain injury. J Cereb Blood Flow Metab 2006; 26: 771–76.

[73] Qiu W, Zhang Y, Sheng H, Zhang J, Wang W, Liu W, Chen K, Zhou J, Xu Z (2007) Effects of therapeutic mild hypothermia on patients with severe traumatic brain injury after craniotomy. J Crit Care 22: 229–36.

[74] Sahuquillo J, Pérez-Bárcena J, Biestro A, Zavala E, Merino MA, Vilalta A, Poca MA, Garnacho A, Adalia R, Homar J, LLompart-Pou JA (2009) Intravascular cooling for rapid induction of moderate hypothermia in severely head-injured patients: results of a multicenter study (IntraCool). Intensive Care Med 35:890–898.

[75] Narayan RK, Kishore PR, Becker DP, Ward JD, Enas GG, Greenberg RP, Domingues Da Silva A, Lipper MH, Choi SC, Mayhall CG, Lutz HA 3rd, Young HF (1982) Intracranial pressure: to monitor or not to monitor? A review of our experience with severe head injury. J Neurosurg 56: 650–659.

[76] Lundberg N, Troupp H, Lorin H (1965) Continuous recording of the ventricular-fluid pressure in patients with severe acute traumatic brain injury. A preliminary report. J Neurosurg 22:581–590.

[77] Marshall LF, Smith RW, Shapiro HM (1979) The outcome with aggressive treatment in severe head injuries. Part I: the significance of intracranial pressure monitoring. J Neurosurg 50:20–25.

[78] Narayan RK, Greenberg RP, Miller JD, Enas GG, Choi SC, Kishore PR, Selhorst JB, Lutz HA 3rd, Becker DP (1981) Improved confidence of outcome prediction in severe head injury. A comparative analysis of the clinical examination, multimodality evoked potentials, CT scanning, and intracranial pressure. J Neurosurg 54:751–762.

[79] Eisenberg HM, Frankowski RF, Contant CF, Marshall LF, Walker MD (1988) Highdose barbiturate control of elevated intracranial pressure in patients with severe head injury. J Neurosurg 69: 15–23.

[80] Howells T, Elf K, Jones P, Ronne-Engström E, Piper I, Nilsson P, Andrews P, Enblad P (2005) Pressure reactivity as a guide in the treatment of cerebral perfusion pressure in patients with brain trauma. J Neurosurg 102:311–317.
[81] Saul TG, Ducker TB (1982) Effect of intracranial pressure monitoring and aggressive treatment on mortality in severe head injury. J Neurosurg 56:498–503.
[82] Timofeev I, Kirkpatrick P, Corteen E, Hiler M, Czosnyka M, Menon DK, Pickard JD, Hutchinson PJ (2006) Decompressive craniectomy in traumatic brain injury: outcome following protocol-driven therapy. Acta Neurochir Suppl 96:11–16.
[83] Roberts I (2005) Barbiturates for acute traumatic brain injury. The Cochrane Library Volume 4.
[84] Povlishock JT, Wei EP (2009) Posthypothermic rewarming considerations following traumatic brain injury. J Neurotrauma 26:333–340.
[85] McIntyre LA, Fergusson DA, Hebert PC, Moher D, Hutchison JS (2003) Prolonged therapeutic hypothermia after traumatic brain injury in adults: a systematic review. JAMA 289: 2992–99.
[86] Abella BS, Rhee JW, Huang KN, Vanden Hoek TL, Becker LB (2005) Induced hypothermia is underused after resuscitation from cardiac arrest: A current practice survey. Resuscitation 64:181–186.
[87] Wolfrum S, Radke PW, Pischon T, Willich SN, Schunkert H, Kurowski V (2007) Mild therapeutic hypothermia after cardiac arrest— a nationwide survey on the implementation of the ILCOR guidelines in German intensive care units. Resuscitation 72:207–213.
[88] Hypothermia After Cardiac Arrest Study Group (2002) Mild therapeutic hypothermia to improve the neurologic outcome after cardiac arrest. N Engl J Med 346:549 –556.
[89] Bernard SA, Gray TW, Buist MD, Jones BM, Silvester W, Gutteridge G, Smith K (2002) Treatment of comatose survivors of out-of-hospital cardiac arrest with induced hypothermia. N Engl J Med 346:557–563.
[90] Holzer M, Bernard SA, Hachimi-Idrissi S, Roine RO, Sterz F, Müllner M (2005) Collaborative Group on Induced Hypothermia for Neuroprotection After Cardiac Arrest. Hypothermia for neuroprotection after cardiac arrest: systematic review and individual patient data meta-analysis. Crit Care Med 33:414–418.
[91] Neumar RW, Nolan JP, Adrie C, Aibiki M, Berg RA, Böttiger BW, Callaway C, Clark RSB, Geocadin RG, Jauch EC, Kern KB, Laurent I, Longstreth WT Jr, Merchant RM, Morley P, Morrison LJ, Nadkarni V, Peberdy MA, Rivers EP, Rodriguez-Nunez A, Sellke FW, Spaulding C, Sunde K, Vanden Hoek T (2008) Post– cardiac arrest syndrome: epidemiology, pathophysiology, treatment, and prognostication: a consensus statement from the International Liaison Committee on Resuscitation (American Heart Association, Australian and New Zealand Council on Resuscitation, European Resuscitation Council, Heart and Stroke Foundation of Canada, InterAmerican Heart Foundation, Resuscitation Council of Asia, and the Resuscitation

Council of Southern Africa); the American Heart Association Emergency Cardiovascular Care Committee; the Council on Cardiovascular Surgery and Anesthesia; the Council on Cardiopulmonary, Perioperative, and Critical Care; the Council on Clinical Cardiology; and the Stroke Council. Circulation 118:2452–2483.

[92] 2005 American Heart Association Guidelines for Cardiopulmonary Resuscitation and Emergency Cardiovascular Care Part 7.5: Postresuscitation Support. Circulation 2005; 112:IV-84–IV- 88.

Section 5

Therapeutic Hypothermia-Acute Liver Failure

Chapter 7

Hypothermia in Acute Liver Failure

Rahul Nanchal and Gagan Kumar

Additional information is available at the end of the chapter

http://dx.doi.org/10.5772/55629

1. Introduction

Acute liver failure (ALF), the manifestation of severe hepatocellular injury in the absence of pre-existing liver disease is a catastrophic and frequently fatal disorder. Though the injury is potentially reversible, the clinical course often culminates in multiple organ failure which is associated with a poor prognosis. The incidence is between 1 and 6 per million population per year [1]. However this data is predominantly from developed countries, data from developing countries where the etiology of ALF is very different is virtually absent. The most common etiologies in the developing world are hepatotrophic viruses (Hepatitis A, B and E) in comparison to drug induced liver failure which predominates in developed countries [2]. Amongst drugs, acetaminophen is the leading cause of acute liver failure and accounts for approximately 50% of the cases in the US [3]. Other etiologies include other viral infections and drugs, ischemic hepatitis, Wilson's disease, autoimmune hepatitis, pregnancy related liver disorders and a large sero-negative cohort where no inciting cause can be identified.

Originally the definition of acute liver failure encompassed the development of coagulopathy and encephalopathy within 8 weeks of the original hepatic insult [4]. Newer definitions differentiate between, hyper-acute, acute and sub-acute liver failure contingent on the time period between the onset of jaundice and the onset of encephalopathy [5]. Regardless of definition used, the onset of hepatic encephalopathy especially Grade III/IV encephalopathy defines a turning point in the clinical course of this disease [6]. Occurrence of hepatic encephalopathy or coma in ALF is a poor prognostic sign and is associated with the development of cerebral edema, intracranial hypertension and subsequent mortality from brain herniation [7]. Though advances in the care of the patient with ALF have led to both a decrease in the incidence and associated mortality of persons developing cerebral edema and intracranial hypertension [7], careful vigilance should be exercised because development and progression of encephalopathy can be rapid and fatal. Further data on the declining incidence and mortality are from a single tertiary care academic center with immediate access to transplantation services. Such expertise may not be readily available at other facilities and therefore the outcomes at such centers could be considerably different. Moreover, cerebral edema and raised intracranial pressure in persons with ALF accounts for substantial mortality (between 25 and 50%) as well as neurocognitive sequalae in survivors.

Given the devastating consequences of development of raised ICP in patients with ALF, it is imperative that early recognition and effective therapies be promptly instituted. Unfortunately prognosis in the absence of liver transplantation is dismal. Medical therapies are frequently utilized to control ICP as bridge to transplant. Often however medical therapies fail to adequately control ICP. Application of induced therapeutic hypothermia has shown promise in controlling ICP when medical therapies have failed. An increasing number of centers have incorporated hypothermia into their armamentarium of therapies to treat raised ICP associated with ALF as a bridge to liver transplant [8]. Emerging data also suggests that this modality of treatment can successfully be used as a strategy to allow for hepatocellular regeneration and bridge patients with ALF and cerebral edema to recovery [9, 10]. Timing of institution, identification of sub groups that benefit and guidelines for use in this condition remain unclear. This aim of this review is to highlight the pathogenesis of cerebral edema and attempt to elucidate the role of hypothermia is patients with ALF.

2. Pathophysiology of cerebral edema and intracranial hypertension in acute liver failure

2.1. Development of cerebral edema

The exact pathophysiological mechanisms responsible for the occurrence of cerebral edema as a devastating complication of ALF are not completely elucidated. Cytotoxic edema appears to be the major mechanism involved in the development of cerebral edema [11, 12], though newer data suggest a role for vasogenic edema as well [13, 14]. Cytotoxic injury secondary to cellular energy failure, impaired cellular metabolism and osmoregulation culminates in swelling of cellular elements and accumulation of water mainly in grey matter. These changes involve astrocytes, microglia and neurons; however astrocyte swelling is a common neuropathological feature of cerebral edema in ALF. Vasogenic edema results as a consequence disruption of the blood brain barrier leading to leakage of plasma into the interstitial space and water accumulation in white matter.

Ammonia is thought to play a central role for cytotoxic injury in this regard and is thought to be the most important factor leading to the formation of brain edema [15]. In animal models, the inhibition of glutamine synthetase, the primary brain enzyme capable of metabolizing free ammonia prevents formation of cerebral edema, despite further increases in brain and plasma ammonia levels [16]. In conditions of acute liver failure, ammonia levels rise in the plasma and astrocytes. In the astrocytes by the process of amidation, ammonia combines with glutamate to produce glutamine, a reaction catalyzed by glutamine synthetase [17]. Accumulation of glutamine along with hyperammonemia in astrocytes leads to osmotic alterations, oxidative stress, changes in the mitochondrial permeability transition, free radical production and alterations in brain glucose metabolism. Together these mechanisms lead to accumulation of brain water and astrocyte swelling [18]. Though the aforementioned cytotoxic mechanisms predominate, an increasing role of vasogenic edema contributing to increased brain water and consequent raised intracranial pressure has been recently recognized. Although structurally normal the blood brain barrier becomes selectively leaky to certain polar molecules through subtle perturbations of the tight junctions [19].

2.2. Cerebral blood flow

Cerebral blood flow is often dysregulated in ALF. Loss of auto-regulation [20] and cerebral hyperemia [21] are two common manifestations of ALF and encephalopathy. Systemic inflammatory response syndrome, particularly tumor necrosis factor has been shown to correlate with development of encephalopathy and raised intracranial pressure [22]. Cerebral hyperemia may also contribute to the development of cerebral edema.

2.3. Raised intracranial pressure

The combination of cerebral edema and increased cerebral blood volume from dysregulated cerebral blood flow lead to increased intracranial pressure in ALF.

2.4. Clinical correlates

Arterial ammonia concentrations greater than 100 umol/L predict the onset of hepatic encephalopathy [23] and concentrations greater than 200 umol/L are associated with the development of intracranial hypertension and subsequent brain herniation [24]. Younger age, development of renal failure, hyponatremia, inflammatory response and the need for hemodynamic support for cardiovascular collapse are additional risk factors associated with the development of intracranial hypertension [24]. Similarly higher cerebral blood flow rates are seen in patients with cerebral edema and intracranial hypertension and are associated with higher mortality [21].

3. The role of hypothermia

A growing body of experimental data and clinical data promotes the concept that induction of mild hypothermia (between 32 and 35 degrees centigrade) is an important therapy in the armamentarium against the development of cerebral edema and intracranial hypertension in fulminant hepatic failure. Hypothermia has been shown to either attenuate or reverse most pathophysiological pathways involved in the development of cerebral edema in ALF.

3.1. Mechanism of hypothermia

In the context of liver injury, hypothermia was first shown to be efficacious in 1962 against the toxicity of acute ammonia loading in mice [25]. Thereafter, Traber et al demonstrated that spontaneous development of hypothermia in a rat model of ALF was associated with significant reductions in both cerebral edema and the time to develop encephalopathy in comparison to rats maintained at normal temperature [26]. This phenomenon has now been demonstrated in a variety of other animal models of ALF [27]. The ability of hypothermia to favorably affect multiple pathways of injury is probably responsible for its remarkable and reproducible effects on reductions of cerebrovascular complications of experimental ALF.

The major explanatory mechanisms for the efficacy of hypothermia probably involve reductions in systemic and brain ammonia concentrations as well as reductions in cerebral blood flow. Nevertheless a variety of systemic and cerebrovascular beneficial effects have been proposed.

3.2. Cerebrovascular effects

Hypothermia, in the absence of changes in circulating concentrations of ammonia, independently causes lowering of brain and cerebrospinal fluid ammonia levels in mice [28]. Hyperammonemia in the brain causes abnormal brain metabolism of glucose, increased glutamine synthesis and increased oxidative stress. Abnormalities in glucose metabolism lead to flux down the glycolytic pathway and increased synthesis of lactate. In an animal model of ALF, inducing hypothermia eliminated the increased lactate and alanine production before decreasing cerebral edema [29]. These observations suggest that hypothermia mitigates abnormalities of glucose metabolism in the brain [30]. Although glutamine has been proposed to be the key metabolite of ammonia metabolism responsible for osmotic disturbances and water accumulation in the brain, prevention of brain edema by hypothermia was not accompanied by reductions in brain glutamine in experimental models of ALF. However other disturbances in other osmolytes such as myo-inositol, taurine, glutamate, lactate and alanine were significantly improved, leading to a better osmotic environment in the brain [28, 29]. Hypothermia in animal models has also lead to the decrement of glutamate and other amino acids in the extracellular compartment of the brain. Brain glutamate is known to increase in both patients [31] and in experimental ALF [32]. Additionally hypothermia has important anti-inflammatory properties. Inflammatory mediators may incrementally enhance the toxicity of ammonia resulting in worsening cerebral edema. Protein and m-RNA markers of a variety of pro-inflammatory cytokines such as IL-1 beta, TNF alpha and IL-6 have been reported to be increased in the brain of rats with hepatic devascularization at the time of cerebral edema [33]. Hypothermia has been associated with the diminution of brain efflux of such cytokines in patients and attenuation of cytokine production and brain edema in animals [34]. Finally reductions in body temperature have led to reduced markers of brain oxidative and nitrosative stress in animal models of ALF [35].

Adverse consequences of ALF on cerebrovascular hemodynamics include increased cerebral blood flow and loss of cerebrovascular auto-regulation. Increases in cerebral blood flow are both absolute as well as relative to cerebral metabolic demand. These alterations play a role in the development of cerebral edema and increased ICP in ALF. Therapeutic hypothermia reverses the increments in cerebral blood flow and restores auto-regulation in patients with

ALF. Hypothermia in patients with cerebral edema and raised ICP refractory to conventional medical therapy not only lowered ICP but also restored cerebrovascular autoregulation to changes in mean arterial pressure and reestablished the vasodilatory response to changes in partial pressure of carbon dioxide [36].

3.3. Systemic effects

Hypothermia consistently lowers circulating ammonia concentrations in humans and in animal models of ALF. In one experimental model, systemic ammonia concentrations were lowered by hypothermia even when hepatic detoxification was bypassed. These observation suggest that production of ammonia is reliant on temperature and that mechanisms of production are perhaps more sensitive to hypothermia than are those involved in detoxification.

ALF is characterized by distributive physiology leading to elevated cardiac output and low systemic vascular resistance [37]. Activation of the systemic inflammatory response syndrome plays a pivotal role in the hemodynamic derangements of ALF [38]. Inflammation acts synergistically with ammonia in the development of high ICP in persons with ALF possibly through modulation of cerebral blood flow [39]. Hypothermia decreases systemic pro-inflammatory cytokines in animal models as well as patients with ALF. Hypothermia also has beneficial effects on systemic hemodynamics; a clinical investigation in persons with ALF and high ICP revealed that induction of hypothermia reduced cardiac output and raised systemic vascular resistance leading to diminished vasopressor requirements [40]. Thus by its potential of affecting both systemic hemodynamics and inflammation, hypothermia attenuates adverse consequences of these derangements on cerebrovascular hemodynamics.

Beneficial Effects	Potential Deleterious Effects
• Improvement in cerebral edema and decreases in intracranial pressure • Decreases in brain ammonia concentration and uptake • Attenuation of brain osmolyte imbalances, oxidative stress and inflammatory markers • Decreases in cerebral blood flow and prevention of cerebral hyperemia • Restoration of cerebral blood flow auto-regulation • Decreases in systemic circulating ammonia concentration and inflammatory markers • Improvements in systemic hemodynamic alterations • Attenuation of deleterious effects of ischemia reperfusion injury to liver • Decreased inter-organ ammonia production and trafficking	• Increases in cerebral blood flow and rebound increases in ICP especially during rewarming phases • Increased risk of infections • Increased risk of bleeding complications • Cardiac arrhythmias • Fluid and electrolyte shifts

Table 1. Brief Summary of the Effects of Hypothermia

Hypothermia may also attenuate liver injury. Hepatoprotective effects of hypothermia have consistently been demonstrated in hepatic ischemia perfusion models [41]. Reductions in metabolic demand, tempering of free radical production, lessening of inflammatory cytokines, preservation of sinusoidal cell function and improvements in the hepatic microcirculation are some of hepatoprotective mechanisms mediated by hypothermia. Similarly in a mouse model of acetaminophen induced liver injury, hypothermia attenuated hepatocyte damage and improved survival [42]. A brief summary of the effects of hypothermia is given in Table 1.

3.4. Clinical correlates

Despite the wealth of animal data, there has never been a randomized control trial of hypothermia for ALF. Most reports are from a single center and have small numbers of patients [9, 10, 36-40, 43, 44]. Jalan et al first reported a series of 7 patients with ALF who underwent hypothermia to control ICP that was refractory to medical therapy [43]. Survival was 75% (3/4) in patients who received a liver transplant while none of those who did not progress to transplant survived. However the 3 patients that were deemed unsuitable for receipt of a liver transplant were only cooled for 8 hours and were then rewarmed to baseline temperature in one hour. The same group of investigators in 2004 reported a series of 14 patients who were awaiting liver transplantation and had cerebral edema with increased ICP refractory to medical therapy. Therapeutic hypothermia was initiated and maintained during the surgical period. Remarkably the survival of this group of patients was 70% and the neurological recovery was reported to be complete [40]. Jalan et al have also reported a series of 16 patients undergoing liver transplantation out of which 5 had high ICP uncontrolled by conventional therapy [44]. The patients with high uncontrolled ICP underwent hypothermia which was maintained during the transplant surgery. Interestingly, all patients transplanted under normothermic conditions developed surges of high ICP during the dissection and reperfusion phases of the surgery related to cerebral hyperemia, whereas, this phenomenon was not observed in the hypothermia group. These observations are encouraging and support the use of therapeutic hypothermia in at least persons who develop cerebral edema as a complication of ALF and have raised ICP unresponsive to medical therapy. However confirmation of benefit requires a well done randomized controlled trial.

The first ever RCT was recently present in abstract form in 2011 [45]. In this trial, Larsen at al. included 54 patients with ALF, in whom a clinical decision for ICP monitoring (imminent brain edema) had been made. Patients were randomized to receive standard therapy or therapeutic hypothermia plus standard therapy. Hypothermia was continued for 3 days. The authors reported no differences in outcomes of mortality, complications or the number of patients who developed high ICP at some point during their clinical course (approximately 50%). Reconciliation of these results, with results of observational studies suggesting major benefit, arises from the fact that persons in this study were randomized to hypothermia prior to the development of uncontrolled intracranial hypertension as a pre-emptive measure. It is prudent to await the final results of this trial to provide important clinical direction in regards to defining the place of hypothermia in ALF.

The previous sections discussed the role of hypothermia in either patients who are candidates for liver transplantation and have high ICP that is poorly responsive to conventional medical therapy or in patients who are at high risk of developing intracranial hypertension associated with ALF. In such persons, hypothermia is used as a bridge to transplant. However, some reports are now emerging that suggest that this therapy maybe potentially be useful as a bridge to recovery in patients who are not candidates for liver transplantation or are at places where organs and/or transplant expertise is unavailable [9]. In previous investigations, rapid rewarming from hypothermia has been uniformly associated with rebound of high ICP, clinical deterioration and death [43]. Therefore instituting hypothermia as a bridge to recovery typically requires prolonged duration of therapy (> 100 hours) till liver recovery occurs and slow rewarming thereafter [9]. It should be the safety and efficacy of hypothermia is this particular group of patients has not been established and the evidence for use is circumspect at best. A summary of clinical studies examining the role and effect of hypothermia in acute liver failure is given in Table 2.

Reference	Description of Study	Outcome
Jalan R et al: Lancet 1999	ALF with refractory elevation of ICP (> 25 mm Hg). Total of 7 patients with 4 listed for transplant. Hypothermia (32-33.5 C) performed for 8-14 hours. Those not suitable for transplant were rewarmed over 1 hour to 37 C. Those suitable for transplant cooled through the transplant procedure	3/3 unsuitable candidates for transplant died after rewarming. 1/4 transplant candidates died. Hypothermia was effective in controlling ICP in all patients and during hypothermia there were no significant relapses of increased ICP
Jalan R et al: Hepatology 2001	ALF with uncontrolled intracranial hypertension. 9 patients were cooled and cerebral hemodynamics were evaluated pre and 4 hours post hypothermia (cerebral blood flow and its auto-regulation, reactivity to carbon dioxide and intracranial pressure)	Hypothermia significantly lowered ICP and cerebral blood flow. Hypothermia restored defective cerebral blood flow auto-regulation and loss of reactivity to carbon dioxide that were observed in all patients pre hypothermia
Jalan R et al: Transplantation 2003	16 patients undergoing liver transplant were studied and divided into three groups pre transplant: Group I - No therapy required for ICP (ICP < 15), Group II - ICP controlled with medical therapy and Group III - ICP uncontrolled by medical therapy and requiring induction of hypothermia pre transplant. Normothermia was maintained during transplant in Groups I and II and hypothermia (median temperature 33.4 C) for the Group III (n=5)	Significant increases in ICP were observed during the dissection and re-perfusion phase of transplant in Groups I and II accompanied by an increase in cerebral blood flow. In Group III neither increases in ICP nor cerebral blood flow were observed.

Reference	Description of Study	Outcome
Jalan R et al: Gastroenterology 2004	14 patients awaiting liver transplantation with increased ICP refractory to medical therapy. Hypothermia (32 – 33 C) performed for a median of 32 hours (range 10 – 118 hours) as a bridge to liver transplant.	13/14 patients successfully bridged to transplant. 1/14 taken of transplant list and subsequently died. Significant decline in ICP within first hour of cooling that was maintained at 24 hours. After transplant 10/13 patients alive at 3 months and had complete neurological recovery.
Jacob et al: Neurocritical care 2009	Single case report of ALF and cerebral edema secondary to acetaminophen toxicity with increased ICP refractory to medical therapy. Hypothermia induced for 5 days as a bridge to liver recovery.	Sustained decrease in ICP with induction of hypothermia that was maintained over the duration of hypothermia. Complete hepatic and neurological recovery reported
Castillo et al: 2009	Single case report of acute liver failure secondary to hepatitis A virus with cerebral edema and elevated ICP refractory to medical therapy. Hypothermia induced for 122 hours as bridge to liver transplant.	Decrease in ICP with successful bridge to and survival after liver transplant
Holena DN et al: American Journal of Critical Care 2012	Single case report of acetaminophen induced ALF who developed cerebral edema and elevated ICP refractory to medical therapy treated with hypothermia as a bridge to liver transplant.	Decrease in ICP with hypothermia, improvement in neurological examination and bridge to liver transplant. Re-transplanted secondary to acute rejection and made complete neurological recovery

Table 2. Clinical Studies Examining the Effect of Therapeutic Hypothermia in Acute Liver Failure

Unlike cardiac arrest several questions about the induction, maintenance and rewarming phases of hypothermia in ALF are unanswered. Though the general principles of adequate sedation, avoidance of shivering, hemodynamic and other organ system monitoring as well as attention to fluid and electrolyte shifts remain the same, there are many issues unique to the patient with ALF. Particularly appropriate patient selection, risks of ICP monitoring, severe coagulopathy in ALF that may potentially be worsened by hypothermia, risks of infection, worsening cardiovascular instability and the potential deleterious effect of hypothermia on liver regeneration are some of the challenges faced by the clinician prior to instituting this therapy. If hypothermia is instituted as a bridge to liver recovery and subsequent resolution cerebral edema, the authors suggest that hypothermia with ICP monitoring be continued till there is evidence of liver recovery and that rewarming proceed at no more than 0.1 degrees centigrade every 2-3 hours.

4. Conclusions

There is a growing body of pre-clinical and clinical literature on the utility of therapeutic hypothermia to control raised ICP associated with ALF. Hypothermia may be used either as a bridge to liver transplant or a bridge to liver recovery. However based on evidence at hand, it can only be recommended for control of intracranial hypertension that is unresponsive to conventional medical therapy. Well-designed clinical investigations are required to clarify the role of hypothermia in ALF.

Author details

Rahul Nanchal and Gagan Kumar
Division of Pulmonary and Critical Care Medicine, Medical College of Wisconsin, Milwaukee, WI, USA

5. References

[1] Bower WA, Johns M, Margolis HS, Williams IT, Bell BP. Population based surveillance for acute liver failure. Am J Gastroenterol 2007; 102 (11), 2459–2463.
[2] Escorsell A, Mas A, de la Mat, M. Acute liver failure in Spain: analysis of 267 cases. Liver Transpl 2007; 13 (10), 1389–1395
[3] Larson AM, Polson J, Fontana RJ, Davern, TJ, Lalani E, Hynan LS et al. Acetaminophen-induced acute liver failure: results of a United States multicenter, prospective study. Hepatology 2007; 42 (6), 1364–1372.
[4] Trey C, Davidson CS. The management of fulminant hepatic failure. Prog. Liver Dis 1970; 3, 282–298
[5] O'Grady JG, Schalm SW, Williams R. Acute liver failure: redefining the syndromes. Lancet 1993; 342, 273–275
[6] O'Grady J, Alexander G, Hayllar K, Williams R. Early indicators of prognosis in fulminant hepatic failure. Gastroenterology 1989; 97, 439–445.
[7] Bernal W, Hall C, Karvellas C, Auzinger G, Sizer E, Wendon J. Arterial ammonia and clinical risk factors for encephalopathy and intracranial hypertension in acute liver failure. Hepatology 2007; 46 (6), 1844–1852.
[8] Raschke RA, Curry SC, Rempe S, Gerkin R, Little E, Manch R, Wong M, Ramos A, Leibowitz AI. Results of a protocol for the management of patients with fulminant liver failure. Crit Care Med 2008 36, 2244–2248.
[9] Jacob S, Khan A, Jacobs ER, Kandiah P, Nanchal, R. Prolonged hypothermia as a bridge to recovery for cerebral edema and intracranial hypertension associated with fulminant hepatic failure. Neurocrit Care 2009; 11, 242–246.
[10] Holena DN, Tolstoy NS, Mills AM, Fox AD, Levine JM. Therapeutic hypothermia for treatment of intractable intracranial hypertension after liver transplantation. Am J Crit Care 2012 Jan; 21(1):72-5.

[11] Kato M, Hughes R, Keays R, Williams R. Electron microscopic study of brain capillaries in cerebral oedema from fulminant hepatic failure. Hepatology 1992; 15, 1060–1066
[12] Ranjan P, Mishra AM, Kale R, Saraswat VA, Gupta RK. Cytotoxic edema is responsible for raised intracranial pressure in fulminant hepatic failure: in vivo demonstration using diffusion-weighted MRI in human subjects. Metab Brain Dis 2005; 20:181–192.
[13] Detry O, De Roover A, Honore P, Meurisse M. Brain edema and intracranial hypertension in fulminant hepatic failure: pathophysiology and management. World J Gastroenterol 2006; 12 (46), 7405–7412
[14] Nguyen JH, Yamamoto S, Steers J, Sevlever D, Lin W, Shimojima N. Matrix metalloproteinase-9 contributes to brain extravasation and edema in fulminant hepatic failure mice. J Hepatol 2006; 44:1105–1114.
[15] Blei AT, Olafsson S, Therrien G, et al. Ammonia-induced brain edema and intracranial hypertension in rats after portacaval anastomosis. Hepatology 1994; 19: 1437–1444
[16] Takahashi H, Koehler RC, Brusilow SW, et al. Inhibition of brain glutamine accumulation prevents cerebral edema in hyperammonemic rats. Am J Physiol 1991; 261: H825–H829
[17] Martinez-Hernandez A, Bell KP, Norenberg MD. Glutamine synthetase: Glial localization in brain. Science 1977; 195: 1356–1358
[18] Vaquero J, Butterworth RF. Mechanisms of brain edema in acute liver failure and impact of novel therapeutic interventions. Neurol Res. 2007 Oct;29(7):683-90
[19] Nguyen JH, Yamamoto S, Steers J, et al. Matrix metalloproteinase- 9 contributes to brain extravasation and edema in fulminant hepatic failure mice. J Hepatol 2006; 44: 1105–14
[20] Larsen FS, Ejlersen E, Hansen BA, et al. Functional loss of cerebral blood flow autoregulation in patients with fulminant hepatic failure. J Hepatol 1995; 23: 212–217
[21] Aggarwal S, Obrist W, Yonas H, Kramer D, Kang Y, Scott V, Planinsic R. Cerebral hemodynamic and metabolic profiles in fulminant hepatic failure: relationship to outcome. Liver Transpl 2005 11, 1353–1360
[22] Wright G, Shawcross D, Olde Damink S, Jalan R. Brain cytokine flux in acute liver failure and its relationship with intracranial hypertension. Metab. Brain Dis 2007. 22 (3–4), 375–388
[23] Bernal W, Hall C, Karvellas C, Auzinger G, Sizer E, Wendon J. Arterial ammonia and clinical risk factors for encephalopathy and intracranial hypertension in acute liver failure. Hepatology 2007; 46 (6), 1844–1852.
[24] Clemmesen J, Larsen F, Kondrup J, Hansen B, Ott P. Cerebral herniation in patients with acute liver failure is correlated with arterial ammonia concentration. Hepatology 1999; 29, 648–653.
[25] Schenker S, Warren KS. Effect of temperature variation on toxicity and metabolism of ammonia in mice. J Lab Clin Med 1962; 60, 291–301
[26] Traber P, DalCanto M, Ganger D, Blei AT. Effect of body temperature on brain edema and encephalopathy in the rat after hepatic devascularization. Gastroenterology 1989; 96, 885–891
[27] Vaquero J. Therapeutic hypothermia in the management of acute liver failure. Neurochem Int. 2012 Jun;60(7):723-35

[28] Rose C, Michalak A, Pannunzio M, Chatauret N, Rambaldi A, Butterworth RF. Mild hypothermia delays the onset of coma and prevents brain edema and extracellular brain glutamate accumulation in rats with acute liver failure. Hepatology 2000; 31, 872–877

[29] Chatauret N, Rose C, Therrien G, Butterworth RF. Mild hypothermia prevents cerebral edema and CSF lactate accumulation in acute liver failure. Metab Brain Dis 2001; 16, 95–102

[30] Chatauret N, Zwingmann C, Rose C, Leibfritz D, Butterworth RF. Effects of hypothermia on brain glucose metabolism in acute liver failure: a H/C nuclear magnetic resonance study Gastroenterology 2003; 125, 815–824.

[31] Tofteng F, Jorgensen L, Hansen BA, Ott, P, Kondrup J, Larsen FS. Cerebral microdialysis in patients with fulminant hepatic failure. Hepatology 2002; 36, 1333–1340

[32] Michalak A, Rose C, Butterworth J, Butterworth RF. Neuroactive amino acids and glutamate (NMDA) receptors in frontal cortex of rats with experimental acute liver failure. Hepatology 1996; 24, 908–913

[33] Jiang W, Desjardins P, Butterworth RF. Cerebral inflammation contributes to encephalopathy and brain edema in acute liver failure: protective effect of minocycline. J Neurochem 2009; 109, 485–493

[34] Jiang W, Desjardins P, Butterworth RF. Direct evidence for central proinflammatory mechanisms in rats with experimental acute liver failure: protective effect of hypothermia. J. Cereb Blood Flow Metab 2009; 29, 944–952.

[35] Jiang W, Desjardins P, Butterworth RF. Hypothermia attenuate oxidative/nitrosative stress, encephalopathy and brain edema in acute (ischemic) liver failure. Neurochem Int 2009; 55, 124–128

[36] Jalan R, Olde Damink SW, Deutz NE, Hayes PC, Lee A. Restoration of cerebral blood flow autoregulation and reactivity to carbon dioxide in acute liver failure by moderate hypothermia. Hepatology 2001; 34, 50–54.

[37] Ellis A, Wendon J. Circulatory, respiratory, cerebral, and renal derangements in acute liver failure: pathophysiology and management. Semin Liver Dis 1996; 16, 379–388.

[38] Rolando N, Wade J, Davalos M, Wendon J, Philpott-Howard J, Williams, R. The systemic inflammatory response syndrome in acute liver failure. Hepatology 2000; 32, 734–739

[39] Jalan R, Williams R. The inflammatory basis of intracranial hypertension in acute liver failure. J Hepatol. 2001 Jun;34(6):940-2

[40] Jalan R, Olde Damink SW, Deutz NE, Hayes PC, Lee A. Moderate hypothermia in patients with acute liver failure and uncontrolled intracranial hypertension. Gastroenterology 2004; 127, 1338–1346

[41] Kuboki S, Okaya T, Schuster R, Blanchard J, Denenberg A, Wong HR, Lentsch AB. Hepatocyte NF-kappaB activation is hepatoprotective during ischemia-reperfusion injury and is augmented by ischemic hypothermia. Am J Physiol Gastrointest Liver Physiol 2007; 292, G201–G207

[42] Vaquero J, Belanger M, James L, Herrero R, Desjardins P, Cote J, Blei, AT, Butterworth RF. Mild hypothermia attenuates liver injury and improves survival in mice with acetaminophen toxicity. Gastroenterology 2007; 132, 372–383

[43] Jalan R, Damink SW, Deutz NE, Lee A, Hayes PC. Moderate hypothermia for uncontrolled intracranial hypertension in acute liver failure. Lancet 1999; 354, 1164–1168

[44] Jalan R, Olde Damink SW, Deutz NE, Davies NA, Garden OJ, Madhavan KK, Hayes PC, Lee A. Moderate hypothermia prevents cerebral hyperemia and increase in intracranial pressure in patients undergoing liver transplantation for acute liver failure. Transplantation 2003; 75, 2034–2039.

[45] Larsen F, Murphy N, Bernal W, Bjerring PN, Hauerberg J, Wendon J, Group E. The prophylactive effect of mild hypothermia to prevent brain edema in patients with acute liver failure: results of a multicenter, randomized, controlled trial. J Hepatol 2011; 54, S26 (Abstract).

Section 6

Therapeutic Hypothermia-Neuroprognostication/Drug Metabolism

Chapter 8

Prognostication in Post Cardiac Arrest Patients Treated with Therapeutic Hypothermia

Ashok Palagiri, Farid Sadaka and Rekha Lakshmanan

Additional information is available at the end of the chapter

http://dx.doi.org/10.5772/55496

1. Introduction

There are over 300,000 out-of-hospital cardiac arrests (OHCA), and 200,000 in-hospital cardiac arrests (IHCA), annually in the U.S. alone. Of these, the survival rate is only 6.4% and 17% respectively (1). Sasson et al. reviewed 75 studies of OHCA, including over 140,000 patients, and found that the pooled survival rate to hospital admission was only 24%, and pooled survival to hospital discharge was only 7.6% (2). Also noted, via the Get With The Guidelines Registry (GWTG-R), was that the rate of survival to hospital discharge after IHCA was 18% for ventricular fibrillation and pulseless ventricular tachycardia, 12% for pulseless electrical activity (PEA), and 13% for asystole (2). During and post cardiac arrest, patients undergo profound systemic ischemia followed by reperfusion. This leads to what is now known as post cardiac arrest syndrome (PCAS), which is comprised of four entities: brain injury, myocardial dysfunction, ischemic/reperfusion response, and the precipitating disease (3). As many as 30% of cardiac arrest survivors will suffer from permanent brain injury (4). The percentage of survivors from the initial cardiac arrest, that subsequently die, is fairly comparable around the world, around 65-75%. Most of these patients die within the first month after return of spontaneous circulation (ROSC). Although the components leading up to survival from cardiac arrest are very important (early access, early CPR, early defibrillation and early advanced care), the main entity that limits ultimate recovery is brain injury from hypoxia. This chapter is mainly concerned with the post cardiac arrest brain injury that occurs and how to prognosticate its recovery. The only treatment that has been proven to improve mortality and neurological outcome is therapeutic hypothermia (TH). Before the utilization of therapeutic hypothermia, many of these post cardiac arrest survivors succumbed to anoxic brain damage (5). As therapeutic hypothermia continues to become standard practice across the world for post cardiac arrest patients, the new question that arises is when and how best to prognosticate both the survivors and non-surviovors of therapeutic hypothermia.Multiple studies have shown that prognostication within 24-48 hrs after rewarming from TH, does not provide reliable resuts (3). In this chapter, we will review the background of prognostication in comatose patients after cardiac arrest, realizing that these recommendations were all made using studies that did not include patients treated with therapeutic hypothermia. It is fundamental to understand the history of prognostication, in order to appreciate the changes that are needed with the advent of therapeutic hypothermia. The remainder of the chapter will review the most recent literature available regarding prognostication of post cardiac arrest victims having undergone therapeutic hypothermia. We will review the utility of the neurological examination, various electroencephalography (EEG) modalities, somatosensory evoked potentials (SSEP's), biomarkers, and bispectral index monitoring for prognostication. Finally we will provide some guidelines for the timeline of prognostication post cardiac arrest and which methods will provide the best results.

2. Prognostication

When we talk about prognostication with regards to comatose survivors post cardiac arrest, we are looking for tools that are both reliable and accurate. In order to help families determine how best to take care of their loved ones, the literature shows that it is difficult to determine which patients will have fully functional outcomes, as this may takes weeks, to months, to years. What is more helpful is to provide families with information regarding situations where there is no chance of functional recovery with data that is fairly robust. With this type of situation, we are looking for studies and modalities that achieve a false positive rate (FPR) equal to or very closely approaching zero (6). It is known that many patients that survive their initial cardiac arrest event tend to have impairment of their consciousness (7). Many, if not all, of these patients require intensive care. Those that sustain the most damage require the most resources. Because of this situation, strain is added to an already frail healthcare system. Thus, it is paramount to develop guidelines that allow for better prognostication post cardiac arrest, in order to guide both physicians and families with regards to appropriate care for their loved ones. Studies have shown that prognostication plays a significant role in withdrawal of life supporting measures for families and physicians. Keeping all this in mind, one must pay attention to the definition of good and bad outcome that each study has chosen to use. In the studies discussed throughout this chapter, most used either the Glasgow Outcome Scale (GOS) or the Glasgow Pittsburgh Cerebral Performance Categories scale (CPC) (see Table 1). Some studies used the modified Rankin Scale. Table 1 differentiates the three outcomes scales. In basic terms, outcome can be broken down into three groups: 1) survival or death, 2) presence or absence of consciousness, and 3) with or without return to normal social activity. Depending on how authors define outcome in their studies, the CPC/GOS categories they use to define 'poor' outcome will vary (8). In many studies, poor outcome ranges between inability to be independent of activities of daily living (ADL) for a few months, to persistent coma/vegetative state, to death (9). Meadow et al. showed that patient.'s chances of survival decreased the longer they stayed in the ICU.Surprisingly, they also found that even in patients with unanimous predictions of death for > 3 days, 12% of patient's survived (10).

	Glasgow Outcome Scale	CPC*	mRS**
Dead	1	5	0
Comatose or Vegetative	2	4	1,2
Severe Disability (Conscious but Disabled)	3	3	3,4
Moderate Disability (Disabled but Independent)	4	2	5
Good Recovery	5	1	6

*cerebral performance category
**modified Rankin Score

Table 1. Glasgow Outcome Scale; CPC*; mRS**

In order to understand the newest prognostication literature, one must have an understanding of from where the current guidelines stem. In 1981, Levy et al. developed an algorithm, which was the mainstay for prognostication for many years (11). The algorithm basically assured no chance of good recovery if a patient had absent corneal or pupillary reflexes at any time after cardiac arrest, or motor response no better than extension at 72 hrs post cardiac arrest. The algorithm that Levy et al. provided us with in 1981 was replicated in 2012 by Greer et al. and produced similar results (12). As did Levy et al., Greer et al. collected clinical data on days 0, 1, 3, and 7, on nontraumatic coma patients in the emergency department, neuro ICU, medical ICU and cardiac ICU. These algorithms are fundamental to understanding prognostication and the neurological examination. Both of these studies have shown that the clinical neurological exam is necessary for determining prognosis in nontraumatic coma, however, it would be helpful if these algorithms were specific to therapeutic hypothermia patients. Greer et al. plan to perform a subgroup analysis from their data specific to TH patients, which should shed some light on this area.

The current guidelines being used were produced in 2006 by the American Association of Neurology (AAN) (13). The 25 years between the algorithm of Levy et al. and the 2006 AAN guidelines, provided ample amounts of research studies, most of which suggested that the neuro exam should be complemented by ancillary tests. The AAN guidelines can be summarized as follows: 1) Patients with absent corneal reflexes or absent papillary reflexes, or no better than extension motor responses, 3 days after cardiac arrest, have a poor prognosis, 2) Patients with myoclonus status epilepticus within the first 24 hrs of ROSC have a poor prognosis, 3) Patients with burst suppression on EEG, or generalized epileptiform discharges are predicted to have a poor prognosis, 4) Patients with bilaterally absent N20 response on SSEP's, between 24 to 72 hrs post cardiac arrest, have a poor prognosis, and 5) Patients with serum levels of neuron specific enolase (NSE) > 33 ug/L between 24 to 72 hrs post cardiac arrest have a poor prognosis. Unfortunately, the AAN guidelines were being written at the same time that the landmark TH articles were coming out, thus providing us with guidelines that did not incorporate therapeutic hypothermia.

They did, however, include in the guidelines a recommendation that once hypothermia became standard of care, the guidelines would need revision. There does not appear to be one single criterion that can invariably predict poor prognosis (14). Hence the need exists for a multimodality approach to prognostication. Table 2 summarizes the salient points of the 2006 AAN guidelines for prognostication.

Neuroclinical Exam	
Strong evidence (Level A)	The prognosis is invariably poor in comatose patients with absent pupillary or corneal reflexes, or no better than extensor motor responses, at 3 days after cardiac arrest
Good evidence (Level B)	Myoclonic status epilepticus within 24 hrs of primary circulatory arrest has a poor prognosis
Electrophysiological Studies	
Good evidence (Level B)	Bilaterally absent cortical SSEPs (N20 response) between days 1 to 3, can guide a poor prognosis
Weak evidence (Level C)	Burst suppression or generalized epileptiform discharges on EEG predict poor outcomes but with insufficient accuracy
Biomarkers	
Good evidence (Level B)	Serum NSE levels > 33ug/L at days 1 to 3 post cardiac arrest accurately predict poor outcome
Insufficient evidence	Inadequate data exists to support or refute the use of S100-B or CKBB for prognostic value
Insufficient evidence	Inadequate data exists to support or refute the use of ICP monitoring for prognostic value

Table 2. Summary of 2006 AAN Guidelines for Prediction of Outcome in Comatose Survivors After Cardiopulmonary Resuscitation

Another important aspect regarding many of these prognostication studies entails the 'self-fulfilling' prophecy (14). These trials have a common bias that is often seen in prognosis determining trials, in which early withdrawal of support occurs in patients who present with certain findings that have previously been associated with poor prognosis. This makes it very hard to determine the appropriate amount of time to wait post TH, in order to achieve a FPR of zero for various modalities.

Perman et al. performed a retrospective review of charts from two academic hospitals, and found that more than half of the comatose survivors of cardiac arrest were assigned the prognosis of 'poor' by their physicians (1). It was also shown in this review that there exists a large variation in the timing of determining prognosis and in the modalities used to make this determination. It should also be noted that in this study, the use of the term 'poor' prognosis was found in many patients even before the TH protocol was completed. The placement of the term 'poor' prognosis into a patient's chart can have a domino effect on the opinions of other medical personnel, and should only be used once objective data has been found. This study provides a great example of why specific guidelines regarding timing and modalities for prognostication in post cardiac arrest patients, who have undergone TH, is of paramount importance.

Oddo et al. performed a prospective study looking at clinical criteria that may help predict outcome in comatose survivors of cardiac arrest having received therapeutic hypothermia (15). This study suggested that patients that take longer to regain ROSC after cardiac arrest, even when treated with TH, have worse outcomes. Another smaller study by Wolff et al. found that patients reaching their target temperature quicker, along with those patients who started at a lower temperature, had better short term neurological outcomes post TH. In 2012, a group created the CASPRI (Cardiac Arrest Survival Postresuscitation In-Hospital) score. This group utilized the GWTG-R, and assessed patients that survived IHCA using prearrest CPC scores (16). This study utilized approximately 28,000 patients for the derivation cohort and approximately 14,000 patients for the validation cohort. The CASPRI score utilizes age, initial arrest rhythm, prearrest CPC score, location, duration of resuscitation, and preexisting organ dysfunctions, to predict favorable neurological survival. This simple prediction tool can be used to help facilitate discussions with families, especially in those patients with relatively high scores suggestive of poor outcomes. Unfortunately, this study did not evaluate the use of TH, and hopefully the study can be replicated using only patients that have undergone TH, as that is now the standard of care. This study found that patient factors played little role in outcome, however factors surrounding the cardiac arrest – duration, initial rhythm, and defibrillation time – were very strong predictors of outcome.

Samaniego et al. prospectively studied 85 post cardiac arrest patients, 53 of whom underwent therapeutic hypothermia (17). They found that the patients undergoing TH were more likely to have received sedative agents around the 72 hr post cardiac arrest mark, as opposed to the non-TH patients. Of the six different findings tested, absent corneal reflexes at 72 hrs, no better than extensor posturing at 72 hrs, and peak serum NSE >33 ug/L at any time within 72 hrs, each failed to accurately predict poor outcome. On the other hand, status myoclonus epilepticus within 72 hrs, absence of pupillary response at 72hrs and absence of N20 response after 72 hrs, all accurately predicted poor outcome. It becomes very clear that the amount of medications used to perform TH will also complicate prognostication, since all six findings were able to accurately predict poor outcome in patients that did not receive any sedation. Keeping in mind that TH affects drug metabolism and clearance, Fukokua et al. found that there was a five-fold increase in midazolam levels in TH patients compared to normothermic patients (18). It is also known that propofol concentrations can increase up to 30% in hypothermia treated patients, and fentanyl clearance also decreases significantly. All of this goes to show that one needs to be very mindful of the types and amounts of analgesia, sedation and neuromuscular blockade agents given to TH patients, along with the amount time passing since complete discontinuation of these medications, when attempting to perform prognostication on these patients.

3. Neuro exam

Al Thenayan et al. in 2008 reviewed 282 charts, and found 37 patients that fulfilled the criteria of patients having survived cardiac arrest and having undergone TH(19). They reviewed neuro exam findings for 6 days post cardiac arrest. This study found that motor response no better than extensor posturing at 72 hrs was not a reliable predictor of poor outcome. It also found that while absent corneal reflexes had a FPR of zero, motor responses no better than extension had a FPR of 14%. In 2007, Yannopoulos et al. published a case series of four patients that provided evidence that predictions based on neuro exam alone are insufficient before 72 hrs (20). In their review, these four patients were determined by a board certified neurologist to have poor neurological outcome, at the time of rewarming. At time of discharge, which was over 72 hrs post cardiac arrest, three of the four patients regained full consciousness, and the remaining patient achieved a GCS of 10 (from 6). A retrospective chart review of patients between 2005-2009 by Rittenberger et al. analyzed both TH and non-TH patients, and looked at clinical examination at admission, 24 hrs and 72 hrs post admission (21). The results of this review showed that the neuro exam was definitely not sufficient to make prognostication at 24 hrs. However, at 72 hrs post arrest, the absence of corneal or pupil responses was highly predictive of poor outcome. This was true for both TH and non-TH patients. In the Post-Cardiac Arrest Care 2010 American Heart Association Guidelines for Cardiopulmonary Resuscitation and Emergency Cardiovascular Care (6), it has been written that no study had shown that any neuro examination findings were able to predict poor outcome in less than 24 hrs after cardiac arrest. A review was performed by Oddo et al. in 2011, which discussed various studies and their findings (22). Rossetti et al. showed that TH provided discrepant results with regards to neurological exam findings, when compared to the guidelines suggested by the 2006 AAN paper. In the study by Rossetti et al. there was a FPR of 24% for motor response no better than extension, 4% FPR for absent brainstem reflexes, and 3% FPR for myoclonus. Other studies have also shown FPR's > 0% when looking at motor responses no better than extension. Oddo et al. made recommendations to wait 5-6 days post cardiac arrest and ROSC, before prognostication, as both TH and the medications used during TH can cause elevated FPR's. They also recommended to not rely on motor reactions alone. From the paper by Blondin et al. it was very clear that sedation and neuromuscular blockade used during TH make the clinical exam unreliable (14). Usually these medications are weaned, but some sedatives and analgesia are continued for more than 72 hrs post cardiac arrest. These medications can confound the clinical exam as hypothermia decreases renal and hepatic clearance of these drugs, leading to higher serum levels and prolonged effects. Blondin et al's review paper found that corneal and papillary light reflexes appeared to retain their predictive value at 72 hrs post cardiac arrest in TH patients. Although there are studies that have shown an FPR of 0% when dealing with absent pupillary response at 72 hrs post cardiac arrest with TH there have been cases where patients with absent corneals and poor motor responses did regain consciousness. From the evidence that Blondin et al. reviewed, their recommendations were that absent corneal reflexes and absent pupillary reflexes at 72 hrs are better for poor prognostication, but should not be used alone. They also stated that poor motor response was not effective at predicting poor outcome at 72 hrs. We have now seen that Al Thenayan,

Rossetti, and Blondin et al., agree that the neurological exam alone is not sufficient to reliably prognosticate post cardiac arrest patients treated with TH. On the other hand, Fugate et al. performed a prospective study, which contradicts this viewpoint(23). This study showed that the majority of cardiac arrest survivors (91%), who were treated with hypothermia and regained consciousness, did so within the first three days post cardiac arrest. Of course, when looking closely at the study, the range did vary from two to eight days for regaining of consciousness, which always makes one hesitate to fully prognosticate within a set amount of time. This paper by Fugate et al. does suggest that therapeutic hypothermia does not delay awakening, in cases where there are no confounding variables. When we talk about confounding variables, we are mainly alluding to sedation, analgesia and neuromuscular blockade. It is clearly shown in studies that when sedatives are used in TH, the FPR of poor neurological exams increases. As described earlier, the inclusion of patients in these studies that undergo withdrawal of life sustaining therapies becomes a self fulfilling prophecy, in the sense that delayed awakenings of these specific patients will go unrecognized. With regards to scores that utilize the neuro exam, the mainstay that has been used is the Glasgow coma scale (GCS). Recently, a more comprehensive score has been developed, known as the FOUR score – Full Outline of UnResponsiveness. Fugate et al. utilized this score to determine if it was able to predict outcome in patients after cardiac arrest (24). They assessed both TH and non-TH patients. For all comers in this study, the majority of patients that scored > 8 on their FOUR score, on days 3-5 post cardiac arrest, survived to discharge. They found similar if not better sensitivity and specificity when compared to GCS prognostication.

4. EEG

Walker et al. showed that close to one out of every twelve normothermic comatose ICU patients had nonconvulsive status epilepticus(25). It has also been shown that up to 44% of post cardiac arrest patients can suffer from seizures (26). In a case report by Hovland et al., they described a 53 year old female suffering from an OHCA secondary to STEMI, who underwent TH (27). Almost 90 hrs after admission, and after analgesia, sedation and NMB's were weaned off, the patient exhibited status epilepticus on EEG. After day 17, the patient was able to dress herself. She required multiple AE's during her admission to control her SE, which may have been recognized earlier had continuous EEG monitoring been used. This case report, and other studies, stresses the importance of monitoring post cardiac arrest patients undergoing TH for seizures. Utilizing EEG post cardiac arrest allows us to evaluate how much of the cortex has been damaged. Ongoing brain damage may occur as seizure activity leads to neuronal necrosis and apoptosis. The 2006 AAN guidelines stated that epileptiform complexes on a flat background, burst-suppression pattern with generalized epileptiform activity/periodic, or generalized background suppression less than 20 uV, seen within 3 days of cardiac arrest, predicted poor outcome with a FPR of 3% (22). However, as stated earlier, these guidelines were with respect to patients that had not undergone TH. It should be known that there are a few common EEG findings seen after cardiac arrest (14). These patterns include extremely low voltage, continuous, discontinuous burst-suppression, and electrographic status epilepticus with recurrent epileptiform activity. In addition, the use of TH can also cause very low voltage EEG backgrounds, which may be due in part to neurogenic medications. Of the various coma patterns that can be seen post cardiac arrest, burst-suppression patterns with little or no reactivity carry the worst prognosis (28). Alpha coma patterns can be seen in 10-15% of patients suffering from anoxic brain injury. Another important aspect of the EEG is the reactivity that can be seen when evaluating patients. This reactivity correlates with the activity of the reticular activating system. One can determine reactivity by providing a noxious stimulus and noting the reactivity of the EEG pattern. This aspect of reactivity will be discussed later in the chapter. The American Heart Association has recommended an early one-time EEG or continuous EEG monitoring to look for seizures in TH patients post cardiac arrest. The reason for this is due to clinical seizures being obscured by neuromuscular blockade or high doses of sedatives. It should also be recognized that seizures during TH can be mistaken as shivering (27). Prior animal studies have shown that TH is protective against seizures, and Orlowski et al. (29) and Corry et al. (30) have shown that TH can be used to successfully treat seizures in adult and pediatric patients alike. One of the proposed mechanisms for this protective effect is that hypothermia increases the epileptogenic threshold, making it more difficult for seizures to occur. On the one hand, although therapeutic hypothermia and sedative therapy may protect against seizures, the use of neuromuscular blockade may mask seizures and hamper their diagnosis and treatment (26).

There have been multiple different grading scales proposed with regards to EEG in order to help predict the outcomes of comatose survivors of cardiac arrest (31). Most popular of these was developed in 1965 by Hockaday et al. With this scale, the EEG was divided into 5 distinct grades. The grades were based upon both the dominant frequency of the EEG and whether unfavorable patterns were present. It has since been shown that unfavorable patterns on EEG correlate with poor prognosis. As stated earlier, the patterns seen most frequently to correlate with poor prognosis are burst suppression and electrocerebral silence. Studies have shown that comatose survivors of cardiac arrest, who initially have poor EEG grades, eventually shift to better EEG grades over time. This presents an important component of EEG monitoring, in which the changes are dynamic, and can progress either favorably or unfavorably over time. In the past, one of the most agreed upon poor prognosis EEG patterns, when present greater than 24 hrs post cardiac arrest, was electrocerebral silence. It should be known that this is very difficult to achieve in an ICU setting due to electrical interference from multiple sources. This being said, when electrocerebral silence is present, it is very significant for poor prognosis. Unfortunately, the data regarding electrocerebral silence comes from pre-TH studies.

When evaluating the EEG findings in TH patients, one can divide the patterns into malignant, benign and uncertain (9). When discussing malignant patterns, we are mainly concerned with suppression, burst suppression, nonreactivity, and generalized periodic complexes. The difficulty with using EEG consistently throughout ICU's is the lack of a consistent classification system and the lack of consistency regarding how soon and how frequent EEG's should be performed post cardiac arrest. Many times after anoxic injury, periodic patterns such as periodic lateralized epileptiform discharges (PLEDs) and bilateral independent lateralized epileptiform discharges (BiPLEDs) are seen on EEG (28). It is important to be able to differentiate between these periodic epileptiform patterns and actual seizures, as intensive treatment of seizures can improve patient outcomes. When reviewing the EEG patterns, one must make sure that there are no concomitant medication effects. Sufficient time after cessation of medications should be given before using EEG changes for prognostication. Since as many as 44% of post-cardiac arrest patients can suffer from seizures, it becomes hard to tell whether seizures are the contributing factor of poor prognosis, or if the seizures are markers of irreversibly damaged brains (32). Mani et al. retrospectively looked at 38 comatose post cardiac arrest patients that underwent TH, and found that those patients that exhibited seizures did so within 24 hours. Many of these patients had their seizures during the maintenance phase of TH. The seizures were refractory to treatment and associated with poor short term neurological outcome. From this study, not only did it suggest that early epileptiform activity can help with prognostication of comatose post cardiac arrest patients in the first 24-36 hrs post arrest, but also suggested that early monitoring of these patients for seizure activity is a necessity. It should be noted that the incidence of seizures in post cardiac arrest TH patients is probably underestimated as many of the medications used for TH have antiepileptogenic properties. A small study by Rossetti et al. looked at six patients that developed post anoxic status epilepticus (PSE) after cardiac arrest and treatment with TH, who eventually improved beyond a vegetative state (33). PSE is comprised of prolonged myoclonic or convulsive seizures or nonconvulsive status epilepticus. This study suggested that when these patients retain their brainstem reflexes, cortical SSEP, and background reactivity (will be discussed in later paragraphs), PSE can be associated with improvement beyond a vegetative state. In another study by Legriel et al., 19 out of 51 patients treated with TH exhibited myoclonus (26). As has been reported in the past, patients that are rewarmed too quickly may develop rebound seizures, and this may have been the case in this study. There were also five patients in this study that developed electrographical status epilepticus (ESE), and all five passed away. This is consistent with prior studies showing poor prognosis in patients post TH exhibiting ESE. In these five patients, the ESE was very recalcitrant to antiseizure therapy. Once again, this study provided more evidence that seizures may be masked by medications used with TH, which was most likely neuromuscular blockade in this study.

When using EEG in post cardiac arrest patients treated with TH, the question arises whether to use continuous (cEEG) monitoring versus spot monitoring. A few studies will be discussed that show positive findings in support of continuous monitoring. Cloostermans et al. looked at 56 patients having undergone TH post cardiac arrest (34). They found that of the 29 patients that had poor outcomes, those with CPC scores between 3-5 all died. This study utilized continuous EEG monitoring on the patients, and found that prognostication could be differentiated by analyzing whether the patient had a continuous pattern on the EEG or low voltage, isoelectric, or burst suppression patterns. Those patients that succumbed in this trial did not display continuous patterns on their cEEG. Rossetti et al. looked at 34 post cardiac arrest TH patients receiving cEEG monitoring (35). They found that the survivors in this study, all 19 out of 34, had reactive backgrounds. As stated earlier, this can be elicited with a noxious stimulus during cEEG, and observing the background activity. Nonreactivity of EEG background in this study was predictive of 100% mortality. Rossetti et al. studied 111 consecutive TH treated comatose patients, and found that unreactive EEG background was a strong and independent risk factor for poor prognosis and mortality (5). One important factor that makes this study stand out from others is that it was exempt from the 'self-fulfilling prophecy'. Background EEG reactivity was not part of the decision making process of the physicians managing these patients, thus proving reactivity to be robust prognosticator. What may be of even more use in the era of TH is the use of amplitude integrated EEG (aEEG). aEEG is simple to apply in critical care patients and also easy to learn how to read. Rundgren et al. conducted studies in 2006 and 2010 utilizing aEEG. In 2006, they showed that all patients with continuous pattern on aEEG regained consciousness. Those with mixed patterns (continuous and discontinuous) did not all regain consciousness (36). The 2010 study was a prospective observational study in which they assessed 95 patients treated with TH post cardiac arrest with both EEG and aEEG (37). The underlying need for this study stemmed from previous evidence showing that TH patients often receive sedatives, analgesics, and muscle relaxants, whose effects are prolonged due to TH itself. It is known that TH decreases the metabolic rate of the body and the clearance of these drugs. Because of this effect, TH patients do not have a reliable exam during the first 24-72 hrs post cardiac arrest. In studies that claim to be able to prognosticate based on the neurological exam within the first 24 hrs, one must take into consideration that these patients may have received less neurogenic medications. With the use of these medications in TH patients, as written earlier, clinical seizures may be masked. In this study by Rundgren et al., continuous EEG pattern was defined as a pattern showing continuous cortical activity, with delta and/or theta and/or alpha frequency waveforms in the original EEG. In this study, patients that started out with, or developed into, a continuous EEG pattern had a higher propensity to recover their consciousness. They also found that patients exhibiting a burst suppression pattern at any time during their monitoring were more likely to succumb to death or continue their comatose state. In this study, having or developing a continuous pattern on EEG/aEEG during therapeutic hypothermia has a PPV of 87-91%. The reason flat EEG/aEEG pattern was not associated with a poor prognosis in this study, was due to 3 patients recovering neurological function with flat aEEG patterns. All 22 patients exhibiting burst suppression pattern at any time during their admission on their EEG either remained unconscious or passed away. In this study, ESE was observed in 27% of the patients. It has been described in the literature that postanoxic status epilepticus has mortality rates that are close to 100%. The patients with ESE that recovered consciousness showed that the ESE arose from a continuous background, which possibly suggests that a continuous background portends to a favorable prognosis, even if ESE arises from it. Lastly, myoclonic status epilepticus (MSE) is a common finding post cardiac arrest (14). It appears clinically as either spontaneous or constant myoclonus. Various studies have found conflicting results, with some patients never regaining consciousness after MSE, and others actually regaining consciousness. From these findings, MSE can not be used to invariably predict poor prognosis.

5. SSEP

The second electrophysiological application that has shown usefulness in prognostication for post cardiac arrest TH patients is somatosensory evoked potentials (SSEP). SSEP consists of a series of waveforms and reflects neural structures. SSEP recordings are noninvasive and can be easily recorded at the bedside in ICU settings (38). Normally, SSEP requires a stimulus that provides an ipsilateral thumb twitch. With the use of TH and the concomitant muscle relaxants used, the intensity of the stimulus needs to be stronger, such that an ipsilateral supraclavicular response is elicited, as opposed to the normal ipsilateral thumb twitch. There are three main stimulation 1 sites to elicit SSEP: median nerve at wrist, common peroneal nerve at knee, and posterior tibial nerve at the ankle. Abnormal SSEP's can signify dysfunction at various points along the neural axis, including peripheral nerve, plexus, nerve root, spinal cord, brain stem, thalamocortical projections, and primary somatosensory cortex. With regards to post cardiac arrest brain injury, SSEP's are used to mainly evaluate the latter three. SSEP's are noted by their deflection and their latency, where positive deflection is denoted as P and negative as N. The number following the deflection notation signifies the latency of the evoked potential. When dealing with prognostication, the objective of SSEP is to determine if there will be return of cerebral function. The N20 peak is felt by most to represent the hand area of the somatosensory cortex. It originates in the posterior bank of the central sulcus and is not influenced by drugs and metabolic derangements.

With regards to TH and the median nerve N20 response, more studies are being published each year, proving its utility. Prior to these studies, the AAN guidelines stated that bilateral absence of median nerve N20 response between 24 to 72 hrs post cardiac arrest accurately predicted poor outcomes. In 2010, the AHA post cardiac arrest care guidelines stated the same, for patients greater than 24 hrs post cardiac arrest; however, both of these guidelines were based on non-TH studies. These findings were confirmed by Zandbergen et al. in their own analysis in non-TH patients, from which they recommended that outcome predictions be made at least 72 hrs after onset of coma. (28). In 2000, Rothstein et al. performed a meta-analysis of 16 studies, covering 572 patients (39). Of these, 229 patients had absent N20 responses, and none of them regained wakefulness. Although multiple studies have shown that absent N20 response is associated with poor outcome, it should be noted that the presence of N20 response does not always correlate with arousal from coma (9). Tiainen et al. performed a prospective, randomized controlled trial, looking at 60 patients, which was a substudy of the landmark European Hypothermia After Cardiac Arrest study in 2002 (38). In this small study of 60 patients, SSEP was compared between TH and non-TH patients. It was found that although TH increases the latency of the median nerve SSEP, the N20 SSEP is preserved in TH. Fortunately the cortical N20 response is only abolished at a temperature of 20 degrees Celsius. Leithner et al. retrospectively studied 112 post cardiac arrest patients treated with TH and having undergone SSEP testing (40). The SSEP.'s were recorded 24 hrs post resuscitation, and of the 36 patients that had absent bilateral N20 responses, 35 had poor outcomes. One patient recovered and one patient had barely detectable N20 responses. Both of these patients had good outcomes and recovered their N20 responses, which brings up the issue of when SSEP testing is most appropriate post cardiac arrest. In the patient with absent N20 responses and good outcome, the patient had severely prolonged peripheral SSEP's, that were felt due to the patient's underlying alcoholism and peripheral neuropathy.

It should be noted that the reason for these patients having good outcomes may not be due to truly absent N20 responses, but may be attributed to interobserver variability of SSEP readings, where it may be difficult to truly differentiate between absent and severely reduced responses. In 2009, Bouwes et al. performed a prospective multicenter cohort study to determine if absent N20 response during TH remains absent upon rewarming (41). In this study, poor outcome was defined by a GOS of 1-2. Out of 77 patients studied, 56% had poor outcome, and of the 13 patients with absent N20 responses, all had poor outcomes. 10 of the 13 patients with absent N20 response survived to normothermia, and all ten of them retained the finding of absent N20 responses. This small study suggests that utilizing SSEP testing earlier during the TH process may be helpful in prognosticating for families. Although this small study showed that the absent N20 responses are retained after rewarming, it should also be known that the presence of a median nerve N20 response can be lost after cardiac arrest. This is most likely due to post CPR delayed hypo-perfusion. After cardiac arrest, the cerebral blood flow can drop by as much as 50%, which leads to secondary ischemia and necrosis. Thus, initially present N20 responses may vanish when tested > 24 hrs after cardiac arrest. These issues suggest that repeat SSEP testing should be done on post cardiac arrest patients treated with TH. From the literature that is available with the use of TH, it seems apparent that median nerve N20 SSEP testing is a robust tool in prognostication, but once again, should be used in conjunction with other modalities.

6. Biomarkers

With regards to prognostication and post cardiac arrest patients, there are two biomarkers that have been studied the most – neuron specific enolase (NSE) and S100-B. S-100B is a homodimer protein found in glia and Schwann cells that binds calcium (42). It regulates apoptosis, outgrowth, and differentiation of neurons. S-100B is part of the S-100 calcium binding protein family, whose name is derived from the fact that it is 100% soluble in ammonium sulfate at neutral pH. It is known to induce the release of inflammatory cytokines which propagate brain damage. NSE on the other hand is a gamma gamma isomer of enolase. It is a cytoplasmic enzyme of glycolysis, and is released into the blood stream when brain damage occurs via damage to the blood brain barrier. Based on these properties of these biomarkers, it follows suit that decreasing S-100B levels suggest improved outcome presumably due to decreased release of inflammatory cytokines, and rising NSE levels are suggestive of poor outcome due to larger amounts of brain damage. NSE is the most studied of these two biomarkers. The 2006 AAN guidelines stated that serum levels of NSE > 33 ug/L at days 1 to 3 predicted poor outcome, in non-TH treated patients. Cronberg et al. looked at 111 consecutive TH patients in 2011 and found that all 17 of the patients that did not regain consciousness had a NSE > 33ug/L (43). At the same time, in 2011, Blondin et al. provided a review article of the data available from prognostication studies, showing that with the use of TH, the cutoff levels for NSE varied, and the previously accepted level for 33ug/L was no longer valid (14). TH has been shown to decrease NSE levels, which correlates with improved outcomes. Multiple studies have attempted to find a 'one size fits all' cutoff level for NSE, but have yet to be successful, mainly due to the small number of patients in these studies. Another issue is that NSE levels can be affected by time, laboratory assay, hemolysis, and hypothermia. The one aspect most of these studies have in common is that a rising NSE level in TH patients does correlate with poor prognosis, and may be useful with other modalities to make life support decisions. Wolff et al. showed that patients that had quicker times to achieve goal temperature for TH had lower maximal NSE levels, supporting evidence that has shown that this approach to TH is beneficial to post cardiac arrest patients (44). One study that showed that S-100B may be superior to NSE for prognostication purposes was conducted by Shinozaki et al. in 2009 (42). This multicenter prospective observational study followed blood samples taken immediately after admission, 6hrs post and 24 hrs post cardiac arrest. Bottiger et al. previously showed that post cardiac arrest patients exhibited hourly variation of S100-B (45). Although 80 patients were found eligible for this study, only 45 of them received TH, making this study's conclusions less valid for the current TH atmosphere. What this study showed was that 'poor' outcome patients had rising NSE levels, and steady S100-B levels. Those patients that had 'favorable' outcomes had dropping S100-B levels. Oksanen et al. looked at 90 patients having suffered OHCA due to witnessed ventricular fibrillation, who underwent TH, and found that the formerly accepted cutoff level of < 33ug/L for NSE was only able to predict 'poor' outcome 100% of the time at > 48 hrs post cardiac arrest (46). The cutoff level they found at 24 hrs was higher, 41 ug/L. From the data that this group gathered, they also found that the rise in NSE levels between 24 and 48 hrs could provide a moderate sensitivity for 'poor' prognostication. In 2009, Rundgren et al. studied a group of TH patients for 72 hrs post normothermia and found that a rise of NSE > 2ug/L between hrs 24 and 48 was indicative of poor outcome (47). Almaraz et al. provided a nice review of the current literature available regarding NSE cutoff levels and prognostication (48). They also noticed that there are limited studies available, various factors contribute to difficulty in finding a specific cut-off level for prognostication including different study populations, different definitions of poor outcome, difference in the laboratory assays and the timing of the when the levels are drawn. The range of cut-off values in studies to date range from 25 to 80 ug/L. One of the largest studies to date, by Reisinger et al., which included 227 patients, only had 20 patients that underwent TH, thus making it not applicable to current practices (49). Lastly, it should be known that reasons do exist for falsely elevated NSE levels including any process that destroys cells both intrinsic and extrinsic, as well as seizures (48).

7. Bispectral index

Bispectral index monitoring (BIS) is a processed EEG monitoring tool. It is a statistically based, empirically derived complex parameter that is based on EEG sub parameters. It provides a score between 0-100, where zero is electrocerebral silence and 100 is fully awake. For general anesthesia, the typical goal is 40-60 on BIS monitoring. Stammet et al. looked at 45 patients in 2009 through a prospective, observational, unblinded study, and found that of the 14 patients that had a BIS of zero all had poor CPC scores (50). Although the BIS of zero correlated very well with poor prognosis, there were 16 patients without a BIS of zero, of which 11 died and 6 had poor neurological outcomes. Seder at al in 2010 looked at 83 TH patients, and evaluated both BIS and suppression ratio (51). Suppression ratio (SR) is the amount of isoelectric activity that is present. Poor outcome in this study was defined as a CPC score of 3-5, and patients that had low BIS values along with high SR values were associated with poor outcomes. Lastly, Leary et al. studied post cardiac arrest patients treated with TH after their neuromuscular blockade was in effect, in order to obtain accurate BIS levels (52). BIS values were taken at the initiation of TH, and at 12 and 24 hrs afterwards. Of the 62 patients studied, 16 of them had a BIS of zero within 24 hrs of TH and all 16 died. These studies suggest that for poor prognostication, BIS values of zero may be useful; however more robust studies are needed for validation.

8. Conclusion

As stated earlier, the parameters found in the AAN recommendations from 2006 were all determined in patients that did not undergo TH. From the literature thus far in the post TH era, the optimal timing for prognostication has yet to be fully elucidated. However, the literature reviewed in this chapter should be used as a new baseline regarding when and how to prognosticate post cardiac arrest patients having undergone TH. It must be recognized that drug clearance is reduced at lower core body temperatures. It should also be recognized that during TH, in order to prevent shivering and decrease cerebral metabolic rate, the use of analgesia, sedatives, and paralytics are standard of care and will delay prognostication due to delayed clearance (1). Friberg and Rundgren et al. have suggested that the neurological exam for prognostication post cardiac arrest be supplemented by at least one other modality, and be performed 72 hrs post arrest (53). The AHA guidelines also recommend that a minimum of 72 hrs should transpire post cardiac arrest and return of spontaneous circulation before utilizing any modalities for prognostication in patients having undergone TH (6). Fugate et al. have shown in their studies that a majority of their patients ultimately wake up by day 3, which poses a question regarding the minority of patients that do not awaken (23). How long should one wait post cardiac arrest and post TH before being able to provide accurate prognostication? It would seem that waiting at least 72 hours post rewarming and 72 hours post cessation of any analgesia, sedation, or neuromuscular blocking agents, is a good start, however, as stated in multiple studies thus reviewed, the neurological exam must be accompanied by at least one other modality. EEG has a robust amount of evidence with regard to prognostication in the post cardiac arrest TH patients (27,34,35). It can be safely stated that EEG should be performed as early as possible post cardiac arrest, and electrographical seizures should be treated aggressively (14). The use of aEEG appears to have a solid place in prognostication of TH treated patients, and is simple modality to adopt in the neurocritical care setting (36,37). Biomarkers such as NSE and S-100B, in the post TH era, do not seem to be able to accurately predict outcome consistently, seen with multiple studies having various cutoff levels for prognostication (48). Finally the possibility exists for BIS monitoring to play a role in early prognostication during hypothermia, but more studies are needed at this time to consider this technique standard of care (50-52). A concern that arises with setting specific time limits for prognostication is regarding the case reports of patients that have regained consciousness well over 72 hrs post cardiac arrest. When assessing these case reports, the specifics regarding the modalities that were used for prognostication need to be ascertained, in order to take these case reports at their face value. Making changes in guidelines for prognostication based on case reports and/or studies with small numbers of patients can cause significant strain on the healthcare system with little benefit for the patient and their families. Thus, there still needs to be larger, more robust studies, to validate the optimal timing and the various prognostication modalities discussed in this chapter.

Author details

Ashok Palagiri, Farid Sadaka and Rekha Lakshmanan
Mercy Hospital St Louis, Saint Louis University Hospital, USA

9. References

[1] Perman SM, Kirkpatrick JN, Reitsma AM, Galeski DF et al (2012) Timing of neuroprognostication in postcardiac arrest therapeutic hypothermia. Crit Care Med. 40 (3): 1-6

[2] Nolan JP (2011) Optimizing outcome after cardiac arrest. Current Opinion in Critical Care. 17:520-526

[3] Nolan JP, Soar J (2010) Postresuscitation care: entering a new era. Current Opinion in Critical Care. 16: 216-222

[4] Sanfillippo F, Li Volti G, Ristagno G, Murabito P, Pellis T et al (2010) Clinical biomarkers in brain injury: a lesson from cardiac arrest. Front Biosci. 2(1):623-640

[5] Rossetti AO, Oddo, M, Logroscino, G, Kaplan PW (2010) Prognostication after Cardiac Arrest and Hypothermia A Prospective Study. American Neurological Association. 67 (3): 301-307

[6] Peberdy MA, Callaway CW et al (2010) Part 9: Post-Cardiac Arrest Care 2010 American Heart Association Guidelines for Cardiopulmonary Resuscitation and Emergency Cardiovascular Care. Circulation. 122[suppl 3]:S776-778

[7] Neumar RW, Nolan JP, Adrie C, Aibiki M, Berg RA et al (2008) Post-Cardiac Arrest Syndrome Epidemiology, Pathophysiology, Treatment, Prognostication A Consensus Statement from the International Liaison Committee on Resuscitation. Circulation. 118:2466-2469

[8] Shonixaki K, Oda S, Sadahiro T, Nakamura M, Abe R et al (2009) Serum S-100B is superior to neuron-specific enolast as an early prognostic biomarker for neurological outcome following cardiopulmonary resuscitation. Resuscitation. 80:870-875

[9] Geocadin RG, Eleff SM (2008) Cardiac arrest resuscitation: neurologic prognostication and brain death. Current Opinions in Critical Care. 14:261-268

[10] Meadow W, Pohlman A, Frain L, Ren Y, Kress JP, Teuteberg W, Hall J (2011) Power and limitations of daily prognostication of death in the medical intensive care unit. Crit Care Med. 39(3):474-479
[11] Mayer SA (2011) Outcome prediction after cardiac arrest. Neurology. 77:614-615
[12] Greer DM, Yang J, Scripko PD, Sims JR, Cash S et al (2012) Clinical examination for outcome prediction in nontraumatic coma. Crit Care Med. 40(4):1150-1156
[13] Wijdicks EFM, Hijdra A, Young GB, Bassetti CL, Wiebe S (2006) Practic Parameter: Prediction of outcome in comatose survivors after cardiopulmonary resuscitation (en evidence-based review). American Academy of Neurology. 67:203-210
[14] Blondin NA, Greer, DM (2011) Neurologic Prognosis in Cardiac Arrest Patients Treated with Therapeutic Hypothermia. The Neurologist. 17 (5): 241-248
[15] Oddo M, Ribordy V, Feihl F, Rossetti AO, Schaller MD, Chiolero R, Liaudet L (2008) Early predictors of outcome in comatose survivors of ventricular fibrillation and non-ventricular fibrillation cardiac arrest treated with hypothermia: A prospective study. Crit Care Med. 36(8):2296-2301
[16] Chan PS, Spertus JA, Krumholz HM, Berg RA et al (2012) A Validated Prediction Tool for Initial Survivors of In-Hospital Cardiac Arrest. Arch Intern Med. 172(12):947-953
[17] Samaniego EA, Mlynash M, Caulfield AF, Eyngorn I, Wijman CAC (2011) Sedation Confounds Outcome Prediction in Cardiac Arrest Survivors Treated with Hypothermia. Neurocrit Care. 15:113-119
[18] Fukuoka N, et al. (2004) Biphasic concentration change during continuous midazolam administration in brain-injured patients undergoing therapeutic moderate hypothermia. Resuscitation. 60(2):225-30
[19] Al Thenayan E, Savard M, Sharpe M, Norton L, Young B (2008) Predictors of poor neurologic outcome after induced mild hypothermia following cardiac arrest. Neurology. 71: 1535-1537
[20] Yannopoulos D, Kotsifas K, Aufderheide TP, et al (2007) Cardiac arrest, mild therapeutic hypothermia, and unanticipated cerebral recovery. Neurologist. 71:1535-1537
[21] Rittenberger JC, Sangl J, Wheeler M, Guyette FX, Callaway CW (2010) Association between clinical exam and outcome after cardiac arrest. Resuscitation. 81: 1128-1132
[22] Oddo M, Rossetti AO (2011) Predicting neurological outcome after cardiac arrest. Current Opinion in Critical Care. 17:254-259
[23] Fugate JE, Wijdicks EFM, White RD, Rabinstein AA (2011) Does therapeutic hypothermia affect time to awakening in cardiac arrest survivors? Neurology. 77: 1346-1350
[24] Fugate JE, Rabinstein AA, Claassen DO, White RD, Wijdicks EFM (2010) The FOUR Score Predicts Outcome in Patients after Cardiac Arrest. Neurocrit Care. 13:205-210
[25] Walker MC (2003) Status epilepticus on the intensive care unit. J Neurol. 250:401-406
[26] Legriel S, Bruneel F, Sediri H, Hilly J, Abbosh N, Lagarrigue MH et al (2009) Early EEG Monitoring for Detecting Postanoxic Status Epilepticus during Therapeutic Hypothermia: A Pilot Study. Neurocrit Care. 11: 338-344

[27] Hovland A, Nielsen EW, Kluver J, Salvesen R (2006) EEG should be performed during induced hypothermia. Resuscitation. 68: 143-146

[28] Kaplan PW (2006) Electrophysiological Prognostication and Brain Injury from Cardiac Arrest. Seminars in Neurology. 26(4):403-412

[29] Orlowski JP, Erenbertg G, Lueders H, Cruse RP (1984) Hypothermia and barbiturate coma for refractory status epilepticus. Crit Care Med. 12:367-372

[30] Corry JJ, Dhar R, Murphy T, Diringer MN (2008) Hypothermia for refractory status epilepticus. Neurocrit Care. 9:189-197

[31] Thakor NV (2006) Clinical Neurophysiologic Monitoring and Brain Injury from Cardiac Arrest. Neurologic Clinics. 24:89-106

[32] Mani R, Schmitt SE, Mazer M, Putt ME, Gaieski DF (2012) The frequency and timing of epileptiform activity on continuous electroencephalogram in comatose post-cardiac arrest syndrome patients treated with therapeutic hypothermia. Resuscitation. S116:1-8

[33] Rossetti AO, Oddo M, Liauder L, Kaplan PW (2009) Predictors of awakening from postanoxic status epilepticus after therapeutic hypothermia. Neurology. 72: 744-749

[34] Cloostermans MC, van Meulen FB, Eertman CJ, Hom HW, van Putten MJAM (2012) Continuous electroencephalography monitoring for early prediction of neurological outcome in postanoxic patients after cardiac arrest: A prospective cohort study. Crit Care Med. 40(10):1-9

[35] Rossetti AO, Urbano LA, Delodder F, Kaplan PW, Oddo M (2010) Prognostic value of continuous EEG monitoring during therapeutic hypothermia after cardiac arrest. Critical Care. 14:R173:1-8

[36] Rundgren M, Rosen I, Friberg H (2006) Amplitude integrated EEG (aEEG) predicts outcome after cardiac arrest and induced hypothermia. Intensive Care Med. 32:836-842

[37] Rundgren M, Westhall E, Cronberg T, Rosen I, Friberg H (2010) Continuous amplitude-integrated electroencephalogram predicts outcome in hypothermia-treated cardiac arrest patients. Crit Care Med. 38(9):1838-1844

[38] Tiainen M, Kovala TT, Takkunen OS, Roine RO (2005) Somatasensory and brainstem auditory evoked potentials in cardiac arrest patients treated with hypothermia. Crit Care Med. 33(8):1736-1740

[39] Rothstein TL (2000) The role of evoked potentials in anoxic-ischemic coma and severe brain trauma. J Clin Neurophysiol. 17:486-497

[40] Leithner C, Ploner CJ, Hasper D, Storm C (2010) Does hypothermia influence the predictive value of bilateral absent N20 after cardiac arrest? Neurology. 71:965-969

[41] Bouwes A, Binnekade JM, Zandstra DF, Koelman JHTM, van Schaik IN, Hijdra A, Horn J (2009) Somatosensory evoked potentials during mild hypothermia after cardiopulmonary resuscitation. Neurology. 73:1457-1461

[42] Shinozaki K, Oda S, Sadahiro T, Nakamura M, Abe R et al (2009) Serum S-100B is superior to neuron-specific enolast as an early prognostic biomarker for neurological outcome following cardiopulmonary resuscitation. Resuscitation. 80:870-875

[43] Cronberg T, Rundgren M, Westhall E, Englund E, Siemund R et al (2011) Neuron-specific enolase correlates with other prognostic markers after cardiac arrest. Neurology. 77(7):623-630

[44] Wolff B, Machill K, Schumacher D, Schulzki I, Werner D (2009) Early achievement of mild therapeutic hypothermia and the neurologic outcome after cardiac arrest. International Journal of Cardiology. 133:223-228

[45] Bottiger BW, Mobes S, Glatzer R, et al. (2001) Astroglial protein S-100 is an early and sensitive marker of hypoxic brain damage and outcome after cardiac arrest in humans. Circulation. 103:2694-2698

[46] Oksanen T, Tiainen M, Skrifvars MB, Varpula T, Kuitunen A et al (2009) Predicitive power of serum NSE and OHCA score regarding 6-month neurologic outcome after out-of-hospital ventricular fibrillation and therapeutic hypothermia. Resuscitation. 80:165-170

[47] Rundgren M, Karlsson T, Nielsen N, et al. (2009) Neuron specific enolase and S-100B as predictors of outcome after cardiac arrest and induced hypothermia. Resuscitation. 80:784-789

[48] Almaraz AC, Bobrow BJ, Wingerchuk DM, Wellik KE, Demaerschalk BM (2009) Serum Neuron Specific Enolase to Predict Neurological Outcome After Cardiopulmonary Resuscitation. The Neurologist. 15(1):44-48

[49] Reisinger J, Hollinger K, Wolfgang L, et al. (2007) Prediction of neurological outcome after cardiopulmonary resuscitation by serial determination of serum neuron-specific enolase. Eur Heart J. 28:52-58

[50] Stammet P, Were C, Mertens L, Lorang C, Hemmer M (2009) Bispectral index (BIS) helps predicting bad neurological outcome in comatose survivors after cardiac arrest and induced therapeutic hypothermia. Resuscitation. 80:437-442

[51] Seder DB, Fraser GL, Robbins T, Libby L, Riker RR (2010) The bispectral index and suppression ratio are very early predictors of neurological outcome during therapeutic hypothermia after cardiac arrest. Intensive Care Med. 36:281-288

[52] Leary M, Fried DA, Gaieski DF, Merchant RM, Fuchs BD, Kolansky DM, Edelson DP, Abella BS (2010) Neurologic prognostication and bispectral index monitoring after resuscitation from cardiac arrest. Resuscitation. 81:1133-1137

[53] Friberg H, Rundgren M (2008) Prediction of outcome after cardiac arrest and induced hypothermia. Abstr. Circulation. 118:S823

Chapter 9

Therapeutic Hypothermia: Implications on Drug Therapy

Kacey B. Anderson and Samuel M. Poloyac

Additional information is available at the end of the chapter

http://dx.doi.org/10.5772/52667

1. Introduction

1.1. Overview of drug disposition and response in critically ill patients

Therapeutic hypothermia has been growing in use over the past several years. Proven efficacy of therapeutic hypothermia in pediatric hypoxic-ischemic encephalopathy (HIE) patients and adult out-of-hospital cardiac arrest (CA) patients has led to expanding clinical implementation in both large and small hospitals. Furthermore, its use to control intracranial pressure (ICP) in brain injured patients, as well as ongoing experimental studies for a variety of other conditions, have led to increased use of therapeutic hypothermia in the intensive care unit (ICU). With increased implementation comes a growing need to understand the ramifications of therapeutic hypothermia on other important factors of ICU care. One such factor is drug disposition and efficacy changes in the hypothermic patient. Specifically, clinical practitioners have postulated the question, "Should drug doses be altered during or after cooling in patients receiving therapeutic hypothermia?" The purpose of this chapter is to explore this question and present the current understanding of the effects of mild therapeutic hypothermia on the processes of absorption, distribution, metabolism and excretion, as well as provide specific evidence of drugs with altered and unaltered pharmacokinetics.

The question of altered drug disposition and response in patients receiving therapeutic hypothermia is particularly important due to the wide array of drugs used in critically ill patients. Critically ill patients are known to have a high rate of adverse drug events. This high rate of adverse drug events is due, in part, to the plethora of medications used for analgesia/sedation, paralysis, control of seizure activity, blood pressure, treatment of arrhythmias, control of blood clotting, antibiotics, and delirium prevention. Table 1 provides a list and details the pharmacokinetic characteristics of the medications commonly administered to critically ill patients organized by class of compound. From this table, it is clear that many of these drugs have large volumes of distribution, are extensively bound to plasma proteins, and require hepatic metabolism as a primary mechanism of elimination.

2. Physiologic effects of therapeutic hypothermia

Before discussing the specific effects of therapeutic hypothermia on drug disposition and response, it is important to first recognize the general physiologic changes that occur in therapeutic hypothermia patients during induction, maintenance, and rewarming. In a broad sense, therapeutic hypothermia is defined as a core temperature less than 35.0°C. Moreover, there are different degrees of hypothermia which incur a range of neuroprotection and adverse physiologic effects. Hypothermia can be divided based on the degree of cooling and include mild hypothermia, moderate hypothermia, and severe hypothermia. It is generally accepted that mild hypothermia occurs when a subject is cooled to a temperature of 32-34°C whereas moderate hypothermia is at a temperature range of 30 – 32°C. Severe, or "deep" hypothermia, is defined as cooling to a temperature below 30°C. Furthermore, therapeutic hypothermia undergoes different lengths of cooling depending on the subject population. Adult cardiac arrest patients typically undergo therapeutic hypothermia for 24-48 hours, whereas neonates with HIE are cooled for 72 hours. The duration of cooling is largely based on the design of randomized control trials which demonstrated outcome benefits.

Although these temperatures tend to be generally accepted, it is important to note that these categories can be arbitrary across studies and require verification of temperature and duration in the currently published literature. In order to normalize the temperatures discussed in this chapter, we have focused predominately on the effects seen within mild hypothermia (32-34°C), since this is the clinically relevant temperature range that has been proven to afford neuroprotection without adverse physiologic consequences to patients in the ICU.

a. Cardiovascular effects

Hemodynamic Effects: Hypothermia has been linked to changes in myocardial function. Mild hypothermia induces a decrease in heart rate, but produces an overall increase in the contractility of the heart in sedated patients. Systolic function will improve, but diastolic function may decrease. Some patients may experience an increase in blood pressure while others may see no change in blood pressure. Overall, cardiac output will decrease along with the heart rate. However, the subsequent hypothermia-induced decrease in metabolic demand tends to equal or exceed the decrease in cardiac output, thus keeping the balance between supply and demand constant. Generally, cold diuresis occurs early during cooling and is of a relatively short duration.

In some cases, the heart rate may be artificially increased by drugs or external pacing. However, the effect of hypothermia on myocardial contractility has convoluted results under artificial stimulation. Two pre-clinical studies showed that under normothermic conditions an increase in heart rate led to an increase in cardiac output and myocardial contractility. In contrast, when heart rate was increased under mild hypothermic conditions there was a decrease in myocardial contractility. The same results were reported in a clinical study in patients undergoing cardiac surgery. When heart rate was not increased artificially, mild hypothermia improved myocardial contractility. Thus, in most patients heart rate should be allowed to decrease with temperature without any serious adverse complications.

Electrocardiographic Effects: Mild hypothermia has also been associated with abnormal heart rhythms. During cooling, hypothermia causes an increase in plasma norepinephrine levels and activation of the sympathetic nervous system. This leads to constriction of peripheral vessels and a shift of the blood from small, peripheral veins to centrally located veins in the core compartment of the body. Ultimately, this results in an increase in venous return which leads to mild sinus tachycardia. As temperature continues to drop even further below 35˚C, the heart rate begins to slow to a below normal rate eventually leading to what is known as sinus bradycardia. The heart rate will continue to decrease progressively as temperature drops to 33˚C and below. The mechanism behind this is a decrease in the rate of spontaneous depolarization of cardiac cells in combination with prolonged duration of action potentials. These electrocardiogram changes usually do not require treatment and in most cases a patient's heart rate should be allowed to decrease with cooling.

Furthermore, some studies have linked hypothermia to an increased risk for arrhythmias. However, hypothermia-induced arrhythmias generally only apply to moderate to deep hypothermia, particularly when temperatures reach less than 30°C. During deep hypothermia, a patient is at higher risk to develop atrial fibrillation or ventricular fibrillation if temperatures reach as low as 28°C. Since temperatures are maintained at greater than 30°C in the ICU, few cases of hypothermia-induced arrhythmias have been observed in clinical trials evaluating the safety of mild therapeutic hypothermia.

b. Renal effects

Therapeutic hypothermia also has physiologic effects on renal function. During cooling, an increase in urinary output, known as cold diuresis, may occur. Cold diuresis results from a combination of an increase in venous return, a decrease in antidiuretic hormone, tubular dysfunction, and decreased levels of antidiuretic hormone and renal antidiuretic hormone receptor levels.

Renal elimination can be divided into passive filtration, active tubular secretion and active tubular reabsorption. Passive glomerular filtration does not seem to be affected by therapeutic hypothermia. One clinical study investigated the effects of mild hypothermia on renal filtration by measuring serum creatinine levels and creatinine clearance in subjects with and without hypothermic treatment. The study found no change in creatinine clearance between the two groups and concluded that cooling does not impair renal filtration.

Although passive processes of renal filtration do not seem to be significantly altered, some published evidence does suggest that the active processes of tubular secretion and reabsorption may be altered by mild hypothermia. To date, the effect of therapeutic hypothermia on the active process of tubular secretion has only been studied preclinically in rats. This study used fluorescein isothiocyanate (FITC)-dextran to measure glomerular filtration and phenolsulfonphthalein (PSP) to measure renal tubular secretion in mildly hypothermic versus normothermic rats. The results showed no change in FITC-dextran clearance, but a significant change in the renal clearance of PSP. These results provide further evidence that the passive process of renal filtration is unaffected by mild hypothermia, whereas, active renal tubular secretion is decreased during cooling. There are, however, a limited number of studies published to date and whether or not these initial evaluations remain true clinically will depend on more extensive assessments of the effects of mild hypothermia on renal drug elimination processes.

c. Electrolyte effects

Therapeutic hypothermia also alters electrolyte levels such as magnesium, potassium, and phosphate. During cooling, electrolytes shift from the bloodstream to the intracellular compartment. The low level of electrolytes remaining in the bloodstream increases a patients risk for hypokalemia. During rewarming, the opposite effect is seen and potassium, as well as other electrolytes, is released back into the bloodstream from the intracellular compartment. If the patient is rewarmed too quickly, potassium levels will increase abruptly in the bloodstream and the patient may become hyperkalemic. To avoid hyperkalemia, a slow and consistent rewarming period is necessary to allow the kidneys to excrete the excess potassium. Furthermore, frequent lab electrolyte assessments are needed to account for shifts in systemic electrolyte concentrations.

d. Body metabolism & drug clearance effects

Hypothermia has been shown to decrease the metabolic rate by approximately 8% per 1°C drop in body temperature. A similar decrease in oxygen consumption and carbon dioxide production is observed. This decrease in metabolic rate arises from a global decrease in the rate of drug metabolism by the liver because the majority of the metabolic reactions in the liver are enzyme-mediated. The rate of these enzyme-mediated reactions is highly temperature sensitive; thus the rate of these reactions is significantly slowed during hypothermia. Hypothermia-induced reductions in clearance have been shown for a number of commonly used ICU sedatives such as propofol; opiates such as fentanyl and morphine; midazolam; neuromuscular blocking agents such as vecuronium and rocuronium; and other drugs such as phenytoin (Refer to Table 1). The specific alterations in drug metabolism and clearance will be further addressed in the upcoming sections of this chapter.

e. Gastrointestinal effects

Gastrointestinal (GI) motility decreases with mild hypothermia. In some cases, decreased motility leads to mild ileus which typically occurs at temperatures less than 32°C. Other physiological factors play a large role in the extent to which drugs and nutrients are absorbed across the gut wall. As with drug excretion in the kidney, drug absorption across the intestinal membranes depends primarily on passive diffusion with significant contribution by active transport mechanisms for some drugs. Also similar to the kidney, cooling was shown to affect active drug transport via the ABCB1 transporter, more commonly known as P-glycoprotein, *in vitro*. However, no affect of cooling has been reported on passive diffusion, thereby, suggesting that passive processes are unaltered and active drug transport may be impaired during cooling. Further physiological factors that affect absorption include the pH of various biological compartments and the blood flow at the site of absorption. The physiochemical properties of the drug, such as its pKa and lipid solubility, in combination with the compartmental pH, will influence the extent of which the drug will distribute into a given compartment. It is expected that some drugs will have increased absorption while others may have decreased absorption during cooling depending on pH, lipophilicity, and primary site of GI absorption; however, no studies to date have thoroughly evaluated if these anticipated changes occur *in vivo* under mild hypothermic conditions. The effects of hypothermia on drug disposition and response will be further addressed in the next section.

ANALGESICS /SEDATIVE	**Primary Route of Elimination**	**Pathway(s) of Elimination**	**Volume of Distribution**	**Protein Binding**	**Half-life**
Fentanyl	Hepatic: 75%	CYP3A4	4 - 6 L/kg	80-85%	3-12 hrs
Propofol	Hepatic: 90%	CYP2B6/UGT	60 L/kg	95-99%	30-60 mins
Dexmedetomidine	Hepatic: 95%	CYP2A6	118 - 152 L/kg	94%	2-2.67 hrs
Remifentanil	Hepatic: 90%	Metabolized by esterases in blood and tissue	0.35 L/kg	92%	3-10 mins
Midazolam	Hepatic: 63 - 80%	CYP3A4	1 - 3.1 L/kg	95%	1.8-6.4 hrs
Lorazepam	Hepatic: 88%	Conjugation	1.3 L/kg	91%	9-19 hrs
Ketamine	Hepatic	CYP3A4 (major), CYP2B6 & CYP2C9 (minor)	2 - 3 L/kg	47%	2-3 hrs
Morphine	Hepatic: 90%	UGT2B7, CYP2C, CYP3A4	1 - 4.7 L/kg	30-40%	2-3 hrs
PARALYTICS					
Vecuronium	Bile: 30 – 50% Renal: 3 – 35% Hepatic: 15%	CYP3A4	0.2 - 0.4 L/kg	60 - 80%	51-80 mins
Rocuronium	Bile: Extensive Renal: 33% Hepatic: Minimal	CYP2D6/Renal	0.25 L/kg	30%	84-131 mins
Pancuronium	Renal: 50 – 70% Hepatic: 15% Bile: 5 – 10%	Renal elimination & Bile	0.19 L/kg	77-91%	1.5-2.7 hrs
ANTI-ARRYTHMICS					
Lidocaine	Hepatic: 90%	CYP1A2 (major), CYP3A4 (minor)	1.5 L/kg	60-80%	1.5–2.0 hrs

ANALGESICS /SEDATIVE	Primary Route of Elimination	Pathway(s) of Elimination	Volume of Distribution	Protein Binding	Half-life
Amiodarone	Hepatic: Extensive	CYP3A4, CYP2C8	60 L/kg	33-65%	15-142 days
Digoxin	Renal: 55 – 80% Bile: 6 – 8%	glomerular filtration, PGP Transporter	4 - 7 L/kg	25%	36-48 hrs
Diltiazem	Hepatic: Extensive	CYP450s	3 - 13 L/kg	77-93%	3-6.6 hrs
ANTI-HYPERTENSIVE					
Verapamil	Hepatic: 65 – 80%	CYP3A4, CYP2C9/19; PGP Transporter	3.8 L/kg	90%	3-7 hrs
Enalapril	Hepatic: 60 - 70%	Hydrolyzed in liver, OATP/MRP2 Transporter	0.2 – 0.4 L/kg	50-60%	11 hrs
Metoprolol	Hepatic: 95%	CYP2D6	5.6 L/kg	15%	3-7 hrs
Valsartan	Feces: 83% Hepatic: 7-13%	Primarily excreted as unchanged drug; OATP/MRP2 Transporter	17 L/kg	95%	6 hrs
Pressors and Iontropes					
Epinephrine	Hepatic & other tissues	Metabolized by MAO & COMT	N/D	N/D	2 mins
Norepinephrine	Hepatic & other tissues	Metabolized by MAO & COMT	N/D	N/D	2 mins
Phenylephrine	GI Tract: Extensive	Metabolized by MAO & sulfotransferase	40 L/kg	N/D	2-3 hrs
Milrinone	Renal: 80 - 85%	Primarily excreted as unchanged drug; Active tubular secretion	0.3 - 0.47 L/kg	70%	1-3 hrs
Dopamine	Hepatic: 80%	Metabolized by MAO & COMT	1.8 - 2.5 L/kg	N/D	9 mins
Vasopressin	Hepatic and Renal: Extensive	Metabolized by vasopressinases	N/D	N/D	10-20 mins
ANTI-CONVULSANT					
Phenytoin	Hepatic: Extensive	CYP2C9, CYP2C19; UGT Transporter	0.5 - 1.0 L/kg	90%	7-42 hrs
Phenobarbital	Hepatic	CYP2C9; UGT Transporter	0.5 – 1.9 L/kg	20-45%	2–7 days
Carbamazepine	Hepatic: 72% Feces: 28%	CYP3A4, CYP2C9; PGP/UGT Transporters	0.8 - 2 L/kg	76%	25-65 hrs
Keppra	Renal: 66% Hepatic: minimal	Primarily excreted as unchanged drug; some enzymatic hydrolysis	0.7 L/kg	< 10%	6-8 hrs

ANALGESICS /SEDATIVE	Primary Route of Elimination	Pathway(s) of Elimination	Volume of Distribution	Protein Binding	Half-life
ANTI-PLATELET/ CLOTTING					
Warfarin	Hepatic: 92%	Primarily CYP2C9 but also CYP2C19, CYP1A2, CYP2C8 & CYP3A4	0.14 L/kg	99.5%	20-60 hrs
Heparin	Hepatic	Metabolized by heparinise; cleared via reticuloendothelial system	0.07 L/kg	N/D	1-2 hrs
Dalteparin	Hepatic: extensive	Primarily by desulfation and depolymerization	0.04 – 0.06 L/kg	Low	3-5 hrs
Aspirin	Hepatic	Hydrolyzed by esterases in the liver to active metabolite	0.15 L/kg	50-80%	4.7-9 hrs
Clopidogrel	Hepatic: Extensive	CYP2C19, CYP3A4, CYP1A2 and esterases		98%	6 hrs
Rivaroxaban	Hepatic: Extensive Renal: 36%	CYP3A4/5 & CYP2J2	50 L/kg	92-95%	5-9 hrs
Dabigatran	Hepatic: 80%	esterases and glucuronidation	50-70 L/kg	35%	12-17 hrs
MISCELLANEOUS					
Quetiapine	Hepatic: 70 - 73%	CYP3A4	6 - 14 L/kg	83%	6 hrs
Haloperidol	Hepatic: 50-60% Feces: 15%	Glucuronidation; CYP3A4	9.5 - 21.7 L/kg	90%	18 hrs
Gentamicin	Renal: 80 - 100%	glomerular filtration	0.2 - 0.3 L/kg	<30%	1.5-3 hrs
Piperacillin / Tazobactam	Renal: 70 - 90%	glomerular filtration and tubular secretion	0.18 - 0.3 L/kg	16%	36-80 mins
Vancomycin	Renal: 40 - 100%	glomerular filtration	0.2 - 1.25 L/kg	30-55%	4 – 6 hrs
Pravastatin	Hepatic: Extensive	Extensive first pass extraction by the liver	0.46 L/kg	43-55%	2.6-3.2 hrs
Pantoprazole	Hepatic: 71% Feces: 18%	CYP2C19/CYP3A4	11 - 24 L/kg	98%	1 hr
Famotidine	Renal: 25 - 70%	glomerular filtration and tubular secretion	1 L/kg	15-20%	8-12 hrs
Corticosteroids	Hepatic	CYP3A4	Varies	Varies	Varies

Abbreviations: N/D: not determined; mins: minutes; hrs: hours; PGP: P-glycoprotein; UGT: UDP-galactose transporter; MAO: monoamine oxydase; COMT: catechol-O-methyltransferase; OATP: organic anion transporter; MRP2: Multidrug resistance protein 2.

Table 1. Pharmacokinetic characteristics of commonly used medications in critically ill patients

3. The effects of therapeutic hypothermia on drug pharmacokinetics

In general, hypothermia can affect drug disposition in various ways. We have previously discussed the physiological changes induced by hypothermia. These effects generally include decreases in active transport processes of drug absorption and excretion, no alteration in passive processes of drug disposition, and a general reduction in the overall rate of drug metabolism. Although these are general alterations, it is important to note that each of these alterations have been shown to be drug specific and requires particular evaluations of drug disposition in the cooled patient. In addition, hypothermia is also known to alter the different phases of drug pharmacokinetics. These phases can be broken up into absorption, distribution, metabolism and transport, and excretion. This section will highlight the effect of therapeutic hypothermia on each of these four phases, and the current research in the area. A summary of the current clinical studies on drug disposition is given in Table 2. In addition, Figure 1 summarizes the known physiologic and drug disposition effects of hypothermia and provides a statement of the level of evidence that currently exists in the published literature.

a. Drug absorption effects

Most drugs in the ICU are administered intravenously. However, some drugs are given non-intravenously, typically via oral administration. Drugs that are administered orally are subject to many factors that influence the rate and amount of drug that can be absorbed before it reaches the bloodstream. Some of these factors, such as disintegration and dissolution, are drug dependent and will vary among drugs based on their dosage form (tablet, capsule, etc) as well as the components that make up the drug (active ingredient, excipients, etc). Physiochemical properties of the drug, such as the pKa, lipophilicity, and solubility, will also influence the total amount of drug absorbed.

As previously addressed in the physiology section, gastrointestinal motility is known to decrease with mild hypothermia. Furthermore, a decrease in temperature can decrease blood flow at the site of absorption, and increase or decrease the gastric and duodenal pH, all factors that will ultimately affect a drug's absorption.

Pre-clinical studies investigated the effects of moderate hypothermia on these physiological factors. Hypothermia is associated with a decrease in passive transport via ABCB1. Results demonstrated a 30-44% decrease in the absorption rate constant, k_a, of pentobarbital, levodopa and uracil. However, these pre-clinical studies induced moderate or severe hypothermia. Therefore, the decrease in drug absorption may be more pronounced than what would be observed clinically under mild hypothermia.

Overall, the effect of hypothermia on drug absorption may lead to a decreased rate and prolonged time to reach maximal concentration for some drugs. Furthermore, the time of onset may be delayed and the magnitude of the pharmacological response, due to these reduced concentrations, may be diminished. However, current studies do not accurately reflect the range of temperature cooling *in vivo* and further clinical studies need to be done to determine if the magnitude of alterations in drug absorption is clinical relevant.

Study Group	Subject Population/ Temperature Cooled	Drug	Route of Elimination	Concentration & PK Parameters
Preclinical Studies				
Tortorici *et al.* [26]	CA rats/30°C	Chlorzoxazone	CYP2E1	↓ CLs, $t_{1/2}$, k_e. ↑ V_d
Koren *et al.* [45]	Piglets/31.6°C	Fentanyl	CYP3A4	↑ Plasma concentrations, ↓ CLs, ↓ V_d, ↑ half-life,
Bansinath M. *et al.* [38]	Dog/30°C	Morphine	UGT, CYP2C, CYP3A4	↑ Plasma concentrations, ↓ CL 70%,$t_{1/2\beta}$ ↑ 2-fold, V_d↓
Satas S. *et al.* [40]	Hypoxia newborn pig/35°C	Gentamicin	Renal Filtration	No change in CL
Nishida K. *et al.* [19]	Rats/32°C	PSP	Renal Tubular Secretion	Total CL↓ 42%, plasma AUC↑ 2-fold, renal secretion ↓
Jin J *et al.* [39]	In vitro kidney epithelial cell/32°C	Digoxin	Renal Filtration	Direction from B to A ↓ 50%
Clinical Studies				
Fukuoka N. *et al.* [32]	TBI Patients/32-34°C	Midazolam	CYP3A4	Plasma concentration↑, V_d↑ 83%, CL↓, K_e↓
Beaufort A. M. *et al.* [46]	Neurosurgical Patients/30.4°C	Rocuronium	CYP2D6/Renal	CL↓ to 51%
Roka A. *et al.* [37]	HIE Infants/33-34°C	Morphine	UGT, CYP2C, CYP3A4	CL↓
Hostler D. *et al.* [33]	Healthy volunteers/35.5-36.5°C	Midazolam	CYP3A4	CL↓ 11% per degree
Iida Y. *et al.* [25]	Brain Damage Patients/34°C	Phenytoin	CYP2C9 & CYP2C19	AUC↑ 180%, CL↓ 67% and K_e↓ 50%
Liu X. *et al.* [20]	HIE Infants/33.5°C	Gentamicin	Renal Filtration	No change in CL
Caldwell J. E. *et al.* [35]	Volunteers/<35, 35-35.9,36-36.9°C	Vecuronium	CYP450s	CL↓ 11.3% per degree

Abbreviations: CL: Systemic clearance; AUC: Area under curve; Ke: Elimination rate; Vd: Volume of distribution; T1/2: Half- life.

Table 2. Summary of the findings of clinical studies evaluating the effects of therapeutic hypothermia on drug disposition.

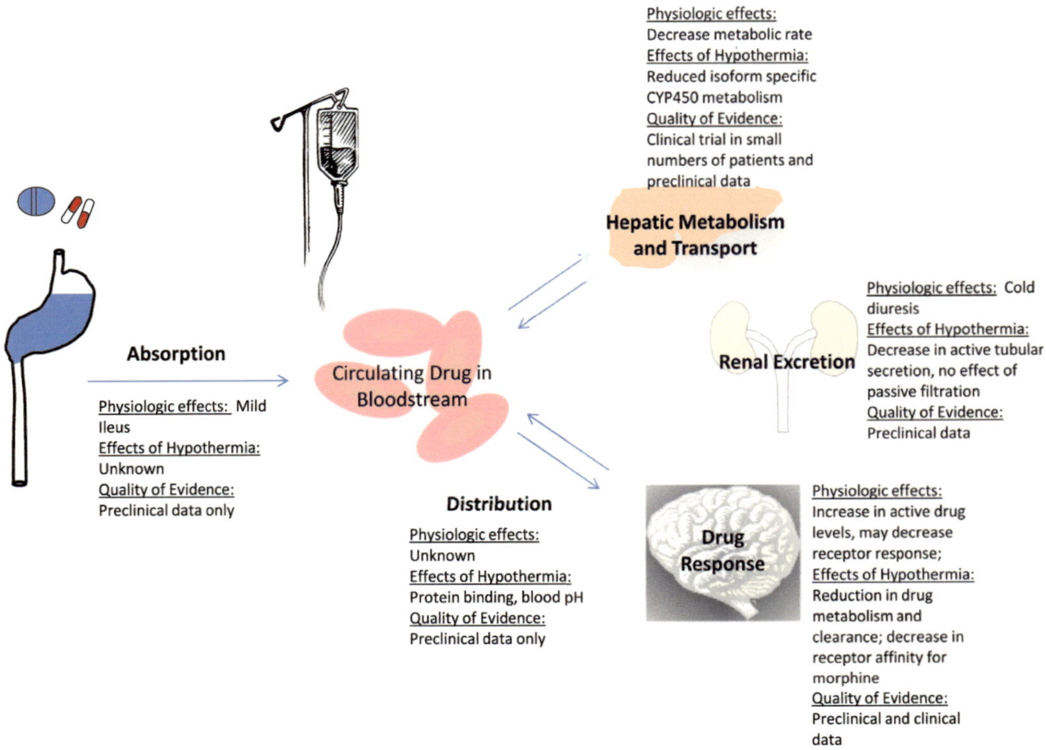

Figure 1. This figure depicts the known effects of therapeutic hypothermia on drug abosrption, distribution, metabolism, excretion and response. Also depicted is the quality of the current data with respect to each of these processes.

b. Drug distribution effects

When a drug is absorbed into the bloodstream, it distributes throughout the body into various tissues and organs. Generally, the space that the drug distributes into the body, or the volume of distribution (V_d), is important for drug dosing since it affects important pharmacokinetic parameters such as the loading dose and the half-life ($t_{1/2}$) of the drug. The factors that influence drug distribution include protein binding, blood pH and lipophilicity. As previously stated, many of the drugs used in the ICU have relatively large volumes of distribution (Table 1), which implies that the drug compounds preferentially distribute into the tissues over the blood. With drugs that have large volumes of distribution it is common for this distribution to first occur into the easily perfused tissues, followed by a more delayed distribution into more difficult to perfuse tissues.

Much of the effect of hypothermia on plasma protein binding is still largely unknown. Two *in vivo* studies (chlorzoxazone in rats and phenytoin in humans) showed unchanged plasma protein binding during hypothermia, whereas *in vitro* studies of sulfanilamide and lidocaine did show changes in the plasma protein binding. Sulfanilamide showed a 65% increase in plasma protein binding when cooled to 17°C while lidocaine showed a 24% decrease in plasma protein binding when cooled to 24°C [50]. A possible explanation for the discrepancy between *in vitro* and *in vivo* results could be the difference in cooling temperature. The *in vitro* studies cool to a much lower temperature than is possible *in vivo* (17˚C and 24˚C versus 31˚C) and therefore may demonstrate a greater change in protein binding. To date, studies have not reported altered protein binding over the mild therapeutic hypothermia temperature range.

Another factor that is influenced by hypothermia is the pH of the blood. As temperature decreases, the partial pressure of carbon dioxide decreases and the pH increases. For every 10 degree change in temperature, the blood pH increases from 7.40 to 7.55. Depending on the pKa of the drug, more or less of the drug will be ionized after the shift in pH. Consequently, more or less of the drug will be able to pass through permeable membranes. Theroretically, drugs like Lidocaine (pKa 7.9) that have a pKa between 7 and 8 may be most susceptible by these slight changes in blood pH [50]. *In vivo* cooling is usually no more than a 6 - 7˚C change. Thus, blood pH would be expected to change in small increments and the clinical effects of these changes remain to be elucidated.

Finally, hypothermia may alter the lipid solubility and tissue binding of drugs. Preliminary studies demonstrate that hypothermia induced a decrease in transfer processes in water/n-octanol systems of atenolol and pindolol. Furthermore, phenytoin was shown to have increased tissue binding in rats at higher temperatures potentially due to temperature-mediated changes in protein conformation, leading to an altered tissue binding capacity [50].

Although hypothermia has been shown to have mixed effects on protein binding, blood pH, and lipophilicity at moderate to severe hypothermia, more studies are needed to determine the clinical magnitude and effects during mild hypothermia in patients. A change in any of these factors during mild hypothermia has the potential to alter the V_d of the drug. The limited number of published studies to date suggest no significant alteration in drug disposition during mild cooling, however, only a small number of drugs have been evaluated with respect to changes in distribution.

c. Hepatic drug metabolism

Many drugs that are administered to critically ill patients undergo extensive hepatic metabolism. These drugs are predominately metabolized by cytochrome P (CYP) enzymes. Various isoforms of the CYP450 enzyme family are involved in metabolism to varying degrees. These isoforms include CYP3A, CYP2C9 and CYP2C19, CYP2D6, and CYP2E1. Of these isoforms, CYP3A is one of the most important in hepatic drug metabolism in part due to its broad substrate specificity which allows for it to metabolize a wide range of compounds. Drugs commonly used in the ICU that are metabolized by CYP3A include midazolam, fentanyl, lidocaine, and vecuronium.

Midazolam is a well-known CYP3A4 substrate that has been most extensively studied in therapeutic hypothermia. One clinical study looked at the effect of cooling on midazolam pharmacokinetics in patients with TBI. The normothermic group achieved a steady state concentration of midazolam which was maintained during the 216 hours. Conversely, the hypothermic group never reached a steady state concentration and midazolam concentrations were about five-fold higher than the normothermic group. Further studies by Hostler *et al.* also saw a reduction in the clearance of midazolam during hypothermia. In this study normal, healthy volunteers were infused with cold saline and plasma samples were obtained to determine midazolam levels and clearance. A significant difference was observed in the overall metabolism of midazolam under mild hypothermic conditions. Furthermore, this study determined that midazolam clearance is reduced by 11% per degree Celsius change in temperature. Similarly, another preclinical study reported about a 17% decrease in midazolam clearance at steady state in hypothermic rats versus normothermic rats after cardiac arrest.

Vecuronium, which is given as a muscle relaxant in the ICU, is another CYP3A4 substrate. The effect of hypothermia on vecuronium was studied in healthy human volunteers. Similarly to midazolam, the clearance of vecuronium was also decreased during cooling. Similarly, these studies demonstrated that an 11% reduction in vecuronium clearance is observed per degree Celsius change in body temperature. Furthermore, a preclinical study by Zhou *et al* demonstrated that hypothermia alters CYP3A activity, however the significant changes in CYP450 activity were isoform specific with significant alterations in CYP3A and CYP2E1 with no significant alteration in CYP2D or CYP2C probe metabolism. Collectively, these studies indicate that drugs which rely on CYP3A metabolism have decreased clearance during mild hypothermia, however, the reduced P450 activity appears to be isoform and potentially drug specific.

In addition to CYP450 enzymes, Phase II enzymes also play an important role in the metabolism of many drugs used in critical care. Phase II enzymes include UDP-glucuronosyltransferases (UGT), glutathione S-transferases, methyltransferases, sulfotransferases, and N-acetyltransferases. Of these enzymes, UGT is one of the only studied phase II enzymes and metabolizes a large number of drugs given in the ICU, such as morphine, propofol, phenobarbital, propranolol, aspirin, and acetaminophen. Of these, the effects of hypothermia on morphine have been most extensively studied.

Morphine, a commonly administered analgesic in the ICU, is predominately metabolized by UGT2B7 with almost no metabolism by Phase I enzymes. One study measured morphine concentrations in neonates with hypoxic-ischemic encephalopathy (HIE). This randomized study compared peak serum morphine concentrations in neonates with HIE who were randomly assigned to either a hypothermic or normothermic group. After 72 hours, six of the seven neonates in the hypothermic group had morphine concentrations greater than 300 ng/mL compared to one of six neonates in the normothermic group. Further, the clearance of morphine in the hypothermic group was significantly decreased. As previously mentioned, neonates undergo a longer, 72 hour duration of cooling. A pre-clinical animal study also showed a significant decrease in morphine clearance in the hypothermic model as compared to the normothermic model. These studies demonstrate a reduced clearance of midazolam during cooling. One possible explanation could be a decrease in UGT activity. Additional studies are needed on other UGT substrates to validate these results.

Digoxin is a calcium channel blocker used to treat arrhythmias in the ICU. A pre-clinical study of ABCB1 transport of digoxin showed that during mild hypothermia the rate of active transport was decreased. No difference in passive diffusion or tight junction activity was seen. The same group also studied the ABCB1-mediated transport of quinidine, another antiarrhythmic drug. In this study, no net effect was seen on quinidine transport during cooling. The authors propose that quinidine is also a substrate for the OATP transporter which may have influenced the results of temperature effects. Although these studies indicate that hypothermia may alter the active transport of drugs by ABCB1, further studies need to be completed to determine the *in vivo* relevance of these changes and explore the effects on other drug transporters.

To date, most of the clinical and pre-clinical studies demonstrate a decrease in hepatic metabolism particularly with the CYP enzyme system during therapeutic hypothermia. Although there is a general reduction in drug metabolism, the magnitude of these alterations appears to be pathway specific and therefore, not all hepatically eliminated drugs will have reduced metabolism. In addition, many of these current clinical studies are small and underpowered. Additional studies still need to be performed to determine the extent of hepatic metabolism on drug concentrations and how clinicians can best dose patients receiving therapeutic hypothermia.

d. Renal drug excretion

Renal drug elimination is a common route of elimination for hydrophilic drugs. Renal elimination can be divided into filtration, tubular secretion and reabsorption. Filtration is a passive process, whereas tubular secretion is an active process of renal elimination. To date, few clinical studies exist that investigate the effect of hypothermia on renal drug elimination. A small number of preclinical studies have explored how cooling affects renal filtration and secretion.

Gentamicin is a commonly administered drug in the ICU to treat infections, and predominately eliminated via passive filtration with little to no tubular secretion. Liu *et al.* showed that gentamicin concentrations remained unchanged in hypothermic neonates with HIE compared to normothermic neonates. This demonstrated that the clearance of gentamicin was not changed during mild hypothermia. Another study investigated the pharmacokinetics of gentamicin in piglets during mild hypothermia. They observed no change in gentamicin pharmacokinetics in hypoxic piglets versus normothermic piglets. These combined gentamicin studies coupled with the aforementioned evidence indicating no alterations in creatinine clearance suggest that mild hypothermia does not affect the passive process of renal filtration.

In conclusion, these studies suggest that the passive processes of renal filtration are unaffected by mild hypothermia, whereas the active processes of renal tubular secretion may be decreased. However, these conclusions are based off of a single preclinical study in rats that investigated the active process of tubular secretion (previously discussed in renal physiology section). To accurately assess the effect of hypothermia on renal excretion, further studies in humans are needed.

4. The effects of therapeutic hypothermia on drug response

In addition to the effects of therapeutic hypothermia on drug disposition and pharmacokinetics, hypothermia has also been associated with changes in drug response. The remainder of this section addresses drugs based on their therapeutic class and the current research showing changes in drug response. A summary of the clinical effects of hypothermia on drug response is given in Table 3.

Study Group	Subject population/ Temperature Cooled	Drug	Drug Response & PD Estimates
Heier T. *et al.* [43]	Patients undergoing surgery/34.5°C	Vecuronium	↑Duration of Action PK mediated, ↑Recovery Time
Leslie K. *et al.* [44]	Healthy volunteers/34°C	Atracurium	↑Response, ↑Duration of Action PK mediated
Beaufort A.M. *et al.* [46]	Neurosurgical patients/30.4°C	Rocuronium	↑Duration of Action PK mediated
Liu M. *et al.* [42]	Children/ 34, 31°C	Isoflurane	↓Dose Requirement
Puig M.M. *et al.* [41]	Guinea pig ileum/30°C	Morphine	↓Affinity to receptor
Bansinath M. *et al.* [38]	Dog/30°C	Morphine	↑Hypotension incidence

Table 3. Summary of the findings of clinical studies evaluating the effects of therapeutic hypothermia on drug response.

Analgesics/Sedatives. Medications given for analgesia and sedation are largely hepatically metabolized and are one of the most commonly used class of drugs in the ICU. We previously mentioned in the drug metabolism section that morphine is one of the most extensively studied analgesics and undergoes predominately Phase II enzyme metabolism by UGT2B7. The effect of hypothermia on morphine response was evaluated in a dog model. In the hypothermic group, a significant decrease in mean arterial pressure was observed, whereas no change in mean arterial pressure was seen in the normothermic group. Another *in situ* study measured the potency of morphine in guinea pig ileum. This study saw a decrease in the affinity of morphine for its target μ-receptor when the temperature was decreased from 37°C to 30°C. In addition, this study reported an increase in morphine affinity for its receptor when the temperature was raised from 37°C to 40°C. This study indicates that during cooling, morphine affinity for the μ-receptor is decreased; therefore, it is likely that morphine receptor response would be reduced during hypothermia even though the concentrations of morphine are likely to be elevated due to reduced morphine clearance.

Another study evaluated the effect of hypothermia on the drug response to isoflurane in children. Liu *et al.* noted that the isoflurane requirement in children decreased by 5.1% per degree Celsius. Furthermore, the isoflurane minimum alveolar concentration values decreased from 1.69±0.14% to 1.22±0% at 37°C and 31°C, respectively. The pharmacokinetic properties of isoflurane were not evaluated in this study so the overall pharmacokinetic change relative to the drug response and dosage is not known so it is unclear if these alterations are due to altered pharmacokinetics or pharmacodynamics. Isoflurane is metabolized predominately by

CYP2E1 and preclinical studies have demonstrated reduced CYP2E1 activity in the rat model during hypothermia. Thus, it is reasonable to postulate that the effects on isoflurane are likely due to pharmacokinetics. Future studies should investigate whether a decrease in CYP2E1 activity is responsible for the decrease in isoflurane response.

Paralytics. Drug response for the neuromuscular blocking agent vecuronium has been studied during therapeutic hypothermia. Mild hypothermia increased the duration of action of the second infusion of vecuronium in patients undergoing elective surgery. Another study saw a similar increase in the duration of action of vecuronium in healthy volunteers during mild hypothermia. An increased duration of action was also seen in atracurium during mild hypothermia. In these studies the increase in duration of action was due to increase concentrations of the paralytics due to reduced drug clearance (i.e. pharmacokinetics). No alteration in the pharmacodynamic response was observed under hypothermic conditions. Therefore, unlike morphine response, it appears that the pharmacodynamic response to paralytics is not altered during mild hypothermia.

In summary, therapeutic hypothermia has been shown to affect the drug response of analgesics, sedatives, and paralytics. A reduction in drug metabolism and clearance may explain part of the response change particularly with paralytics. Conversely, a reduced affinity of morphine for the μ-receptor has been reported. Careful pharmacotherapeutic monitoring in the clinic during hypothermia treatment may be necessary to prevent a potential therapy-drug interaction caused by changes in both drug concentration and in drug response during cooling.

5. Prospectus and future directions

Therapeutic hypothermia has been shown to be a beneficial neuroprotective therapy in critical care. In addition to the benefits for therapeutic hypothermia, there are potential side effects that can also occur. The effect of hypothermia on drug metabolism and clearance can lead to elevations in drug concentrations. Recent studies have reported that the effect of hypothermia on drug metabolism and the degree of change can be specific for the metabolism and elimination route. A small number of studies have investigated the effect of hypothermia on drug response including analgesics, sedatives and paralytics. The effect on drug response may be due to pharmacokinetic and pharmacodynamics alterations during hypothermia.

However, the effect of therapeutic hypothermia on drug disposition and response is still significantly understudied. To date, little is still understood as to how therapeutic hypothermia affects the wide array of drugs administered to critically ill patients in the ICU. In order to safely use this therapy in patients, it is imperative that we further evaluate the potential alterations on drug metabolism and response. Larger clinical trials in humans are necessary before we can fully understand the effects of therapeutic hypothermia on drug pharmacokinetics. Ultimately by understanding the physiological effects of hypothermia, awareness of hypothermia's effect on drug pharmacokinetics, and learning the potential side effects, we will be able to more safely and effectively use this neuroprotective strategy in a wide range of critically ill patients.

Author details

Kacey B. Anderson and Samuel M. Poloyac
University of Pittsburgh, School of Pharmacy, Department of Pharmaceutical Sciences, Pittsburgh, PA, USA

6. References

[1] Cullen, D.J., Preventable adverse drug events in hospitalized patients: a comparative study of intensive care and general care units. Critical Care Medicine, 1997. 25(8): p. 1289-1297.

[2] Shankaran S., P.A., McDonald S. A., et al., Childhood Outcomes after Hypothermia for Neonatal Encephalopathy. The New England Journal of Medicine, 2012. 366(22): p. 2085-2092.

[3] Shankaran S., L.A.R., Ehrenkranz R. A., et al Whole-body hypothermia for neonates with hypoxic–ischemic encephalopathy. New England Journal of Medicine, 2005. 353: p. 1574-1584.

[4] Bernard S. A., G.T.W., Buist M. D., et al, Treatment of comatose survivors of out-of-hospital cardiac arrest with induced hypothermia. New England Journal of Medicine, 2002. 34: p. 557-563.

[5] Polderman K.H., H.I., Therapeutic hypothermia and controlled normothermia in the intensive care unit: Practical considerations, side effects and cooling methods. Critical Care Medicine, 2009. 37(3): p. 1101-1120.

[6] Fischer U.M., C.C.S.J., Laine G.A., et al, Mild hypothermia impairs left ventricular diastolic but not systolic function. Journal of Investigative Surgery, 2005. 18: p. 291-296.

[7] L.I., G., Effects of hypothermia on contractility of the intact dog heart. American Journal of Physiology, 1958. 194: p. 92-98.

[8] Suga H, G.Y., Igarashi Y, et al, Cardiac cooling increases Emax without affecting relation between O2 consumption and systolic pressure-volume area in dog left ventricle. Circulation Research, 1988. 63: p. 61-71.

[9] Mikane T., A.J., Suzuki S. et al., O2 cost of contractility but not of mechanical energy increases with temperature in canine left ventricle. American Journal of Physiology, 1999. 277: p. H65-H73.

[10] Lewis M. E., A.-K.A.H., Townend J. N., et al., The effects of hypothermia on human left ventricular contractile function during cardiac surgery. Journal of the American College of Cardiology, 2002. 39: p. 102-108.

[11] Polderman, K.H., Mechanism of action, physiological effects, and complications of hypothermia. Critical Care Medicine, 2009. 37(7): p. 186-202.

[12] Mattheussen M., M.K., Van Aken H. et al., Interaction of heart rate and hypothermia on global myocardial contraction of the isolated rabbit heart. Anesthesia & Analgesia, 1996. 82: p. 975-981.

[13] Danzl D.F., P.R.S., Accidental Hypothermia. New England Journal of Medicine, 1994. 331(26): p. 1756-1760.

[14] Polderman, K.H.P.S.M., Girbes A.R.J., Hypophosphatemia and hypomagnesemia induced by cooling in patients with severe head injury. J Neurosurg, 2001. 94: p. 697-705.

[15] Polderman K.H., T.T.J.R., Peerdeman and e.a. S.M., Effects of artificially induced hypothermia on intracranial pressure and outcome in patients with severe traumatic head injury. Intensive Care Medicine, 2002. 28: p. 1563-1567.
[16] Pozos R.S., D.D., Medical Aspects of Harsh Environments. Human physiological responses to cold stress and hypothermia, ed. P.K.B.a.B. R.E. Vol. 1. 2001, Washington, D.C.: Walter Reed Army Medical Center Borden Institute.
[17] Morgan M.L., A.R.J., Ellis M.A., et al Mechanism of cold diuresis in the rat. American Journal of Physiology, 1983. 244: p. F210-F216.
[18] Allen D.E., G.M., Mechanisms for the diuresis of acute cold exposure: Role for vasopressin? American Journal of Physiology, 1993. 264: p. R524-R532.
[19] Z., S., Genetic AVP deficiency abolishes coldinduced diuresis but does not attenuate coldinduced hypertension American Journal of Physiology Renal Physiology, 2006. 290: p. F1472-F1477.
[20] Sun Z., Z.Z., Cade R., Renal responses to chronic cold exposure Canadian Journal of Physiology and Pharmacology, 2003. 81: p. 22-27.
[21] Zeiner A., S.-P.J., Sterz F., Holzer M., Losert H., Laggner A. N., Mullner M., The effect of mild hypothermia on renal function after cardiopulmonary resuscitation in men. Resuscitation, 2004. 60(3): p. 253-261.
[22] Nishida K., O.M., Sakamoto R., et al., Change in pharmacokinetics of model compounds with different elimination processes in rats during hypothermia. Biological and Pharmaceuticals Bulletin, 2007. 30: p. 1763-1767.
[23] Liu X., B.M., Stone J., et al., Serum gentamicin concentrations in encephalopathic infants are not affected by therapeutic hypothermia. Pediatrics, 2009. 124: p. 310-315.
[24] A., B., Effects of body temperature on blood gases. Intensive Care Medicine, 2005. 31: p. 24-27.
[25] Hernandez, M.A., Rathinavelu, A., Basic Pharmacology: Understanding Drug Actions and Reactions.2006, Florida: CRC Press Pharmacy Education.
[26] Stavchansky S, T.I., Effect of hypothermia on the intestinal absorption of uracil and L-dopa in the rat. Journal of Pharmaceutical Science, 1987. 76(9): p. 688-691.
[27] Stavchansky S, T.I., Effects of hypothermia on drug absorption. Pharmaceutical Research, 1987. 4(3): p. 248-250.
[28] Iida Y., N.S., Asada A., Effect of mild therapeutic hypothermia on phenytoin pharmacokinetics. Therapeutic Drug Monitoring, 2001. 23(3): p. 192-197.
[29] Tortorici M.A., K.P.M., Bies R.R., et al., Therapeutic hypothermiainduced pharmacokinetic alterations on CYP2E1 chlorzoxazone-mediated metabolism in a cardiac arrest rat model. Critical Care Medicine, 2006. 34(3): p. 785-791.
[30] Kalser S.C., K.E.J., Randolph M.M., Drug metabolism in hypothermia: uptake, metabolism and excretion of S35-sulfanilamide by the isolated, perfused rat liver. Journal of Pharmacology and Experimental Therapeutics, 1968. 159(2): p. 389-398.
[31] Lonnqvist P.A., H.L., Plasma protein binding of lidocaine during hypothermic conditions. Perfusion, 1993. 8: p. 221-224.
[32] Groenendaal F., D.V.K.M.K., van Bel F., Blood gas values during hypothermia in asphyxiated term neonates. Pediatrics, 2009. 123: p. 170-172.
[33] Perlovich G.L., V.T.V., Bauer-Brandl A., Thermodynamic study of sublimation, solubility, solvation, and distribution processes of atenolol and pindolol. Molecular Pharmacology, 2007. 4(6): p. 929-935.

[34] Kato Y., H.J., Sakaguchi K., et al., Enhancement of phenytoin binding to tissues in rats by heat treatment. Journal of Pharmacy and Pharmacology, 1989. 41(2): p. 125-126.

[35] Fukuoka N., A.M., Tsukamoto T., et al., Biphasic concentration change during continuous midazolam administration in brain-injured patients undergoing therapeutic moderate hypothermia. Resuscitation, 2004. 60: p. 225-230.

[36] Hostler D., Z.J., Tortorici M.A., et al., Mild hypothermia alters midazolam pharmacokinetics in normal healthy volunteers. Drug Metabolism and Disposition, 2010. 38: p. 781-788.

[37] Zhou J., E.P.E., Bies R. R., Kochanek P. M., Poloyac S.M., Cardiac Arrest and Therapeutic Hypothermia Decrease Isoform-Specific Cytochrome P450 Drug Metabolism. Drug Metabolism and Disposition 2011. 39(12): p. 2209-2218.

[38] Caldwell J. E., H.T., Wright P.M., et al., Temperature-dependent pharmacokinetics and pharmacodynamics of vecuronium. Anesthesiology, 2000. 92: p. 84-93.

[39] Kumar G. N., S.S., Role of drug metabolism in drug discovery and developement. Medical Care Research and Review, 2001. 21: p. 397-411.

[40] Roka A., M.K.T., Vasarhelyi B., et al., Elevated morphine concentrations in neonates treated with morphine and prolonged hypothermia for hypoxic ischemic encephalopathy. Pediatrics, 2008. 121: p. e844-849.

[41] Bansinath M., M.K.T., Vasarhelyi B., et al., Influence of hypo and hyperthermia on disposition of morphine. J of Clinical Pharmacology, 1988. 28: p. 860-864.

[42] Jin J. S., S.T., Kakumoto M, et al., Effect of therapeutic moderate hypothermia on multi-drug resistance protein 1-mediated transepithelial transport of drugs. Neurol Med Chir, 2006. 46: p. 321-327.

[43] Satas S., H.N.O., Melby K., et al., Influence of mild hypothermia after hypoxia-ischemia on the pharmacokinetics of gentamicin in newborn pigs. Biology of the Neonates, 2000. 77: p. 50-57.

[44] Puig M. M., W.W., Tang C. K., et al., Effects of temperature on the interaction of morphine with opioid receptors. British Journal of Anaesthesia, 1987. 35: p. 2196-2204.

[45] Liu M., H.X., Liu J., The effect of hypothermia on isoflurane MAC in children. Anesthesiology, 2001. 94: p. 429-432.

[46] Heier T., C.J.E., Sessler D. I., et al., Mild intraoperative hypothermia increases duration of action and spontaneous recovery of vecuronium blockade during nitrous oxide-isoflurane anesthesia in humans. Anesthesiology, 1991. 74: p. 815-819.

[47] Leslie K., S.D.I., Bjorksten A. R., et al., Mild hypothermia alters propofol pharmacokinetics and increases the duration of action of atracurium. Anesthesia & Analgesia, 1995. 80: p. 1007-1114.

[48] Koren G., B.C., Goresky G., Bohn D., Klein J., MacLeod S. M., Biggar W. D., The influence of hypothermia on the disposition of fentanyl-Human animal studies. European Journal of Clinical Pharmacology 1987. 32: p. 373-376.

[49] Beaufort A.M., W.J.M., Belopavlovic M., et al., The influence of hypothermia (surface cooling) on the time-course of action and on the pharmacokinetics of rocuronium in humans. European Journal of Anaesthesiology, 1995. 11: p. 95-106.

[50] Van den Broek M. P.H., Groenendaal F., Egberts A. C.G., Rademaker C. M. A. Effects of Hypothermia on Pharmacokinetics and Pharmacodynamics. Clinical Pharmacokinetics, 2010. 49 (5): p. 277-294.